Endodontics Manual for the General Dentist

Martin Trope, DMD
J.B. Freedland Professor and Chair
Department of Endodontics
University of North Carolina
Chapel Hill, North Carolina

Gilberto J. Debelian, DMD, PhD
Private Practice
Bekkestua, Norway

Quintessence Publishing Co, Ltd
London, Berlin, Chicago, Paris, Milan, Barcelona, Istanbul,
Saõ Paulo, Tokyo, New Delhi, Moscow, Prague, Warsaw

British Library Cataloguing in Publication Data
Trope, Martin
Endodontics Manual for the General Dentist
1. Endodontics
I. Title II. Debelian, Gilberto
617.6'342

Quintessence Publishing Co, Ltd
Grafton Road
New Malden, Surrey KT3 3AB
United Kingdom
www.quintpub.co.uk

ISBN 1-85097-089-0

Printed in Germany

Table of Contents

Preface

Root canal therapy requires a high level of technical skill. However, without a correct diagnosis and a clear understanding of the biologic fundamentals governing a successful outcome, a clinician's skills may be wasted on complicated techniques or inappropriate treatments. A correct diagnosis, in combination with the right choice of new materials and techniques, will ensure an environment that offers an extremely high probability of success and a healthy apical periodontium. The authors hope that, after reading this manual, you will find the practice of endodontics simple—and predictably successful.

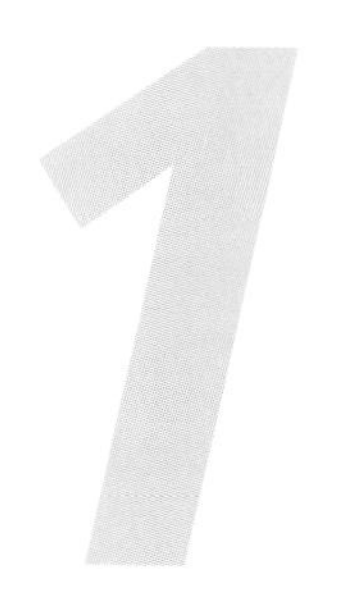

Introduction to Endodontics

Before proceeding to the specifics of endodontic treatment, it is extremely important for the dentist to have a clear understanding of the *clinical* definition of endodontics. As part of the health care profession, each dental specialty needs to be focused on a specific disease. For endodontics, the disease of interest is *apical periodontitis*—periodontal attachment inflammation at the apex of the tooth. In rare cases, periodontitis of endodontic origin may be located in a position other than the apex of the tooth; these cases are described as *peri-radicular periodontitis*. Apical periodontitis manifests as pain originating from the apical periodontium or, more commonly, as (pain-free) radiolucency on the radiograph (Fig 1-1). Histologically, it resembles a granuloma or cyst (Fig 1-2).

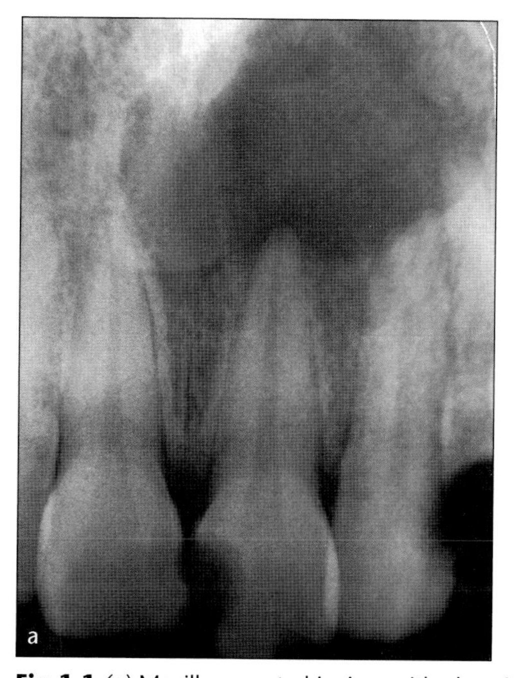

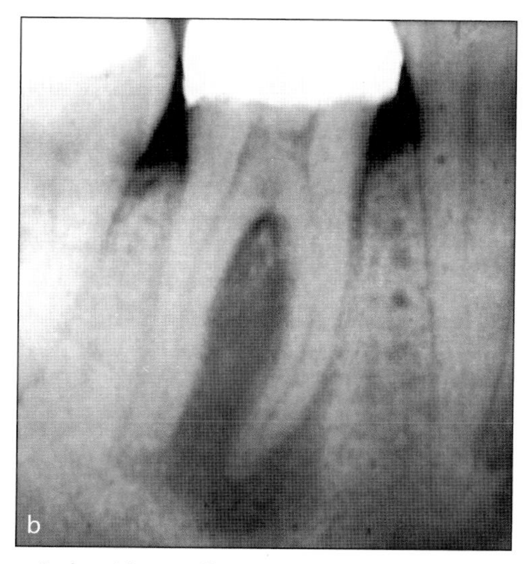

Fig 1-1 *(a)* Maxillary central incisor with chronic periodontitis manifesting as a radiolucency. *(b)* Mandibular molar with radiolucency typical of periradicular periodontitis.

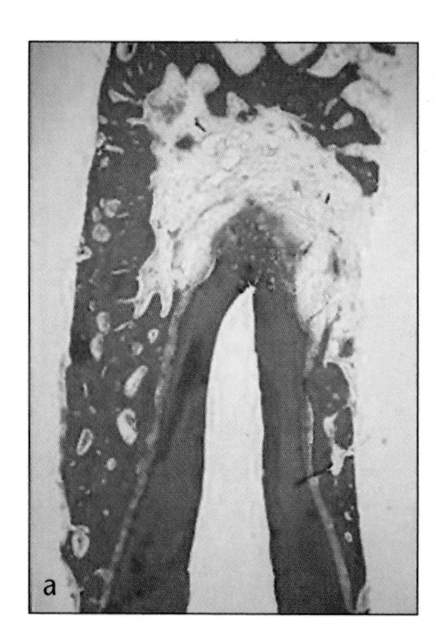

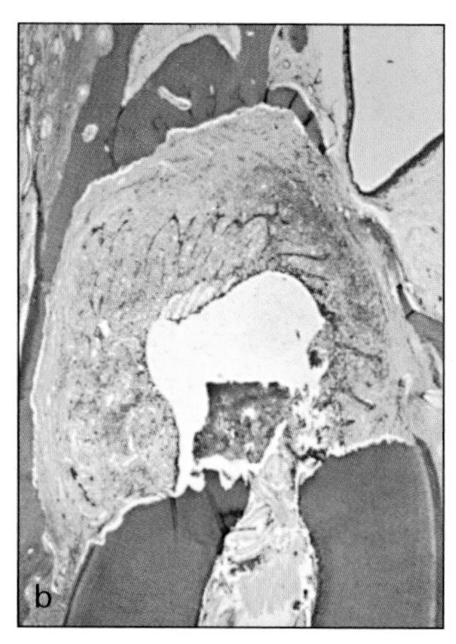

Fig 1-2 Histologically, a periapical lesion will sometimes appear as *(a)* a granuloma, or *(b)* a cyst.

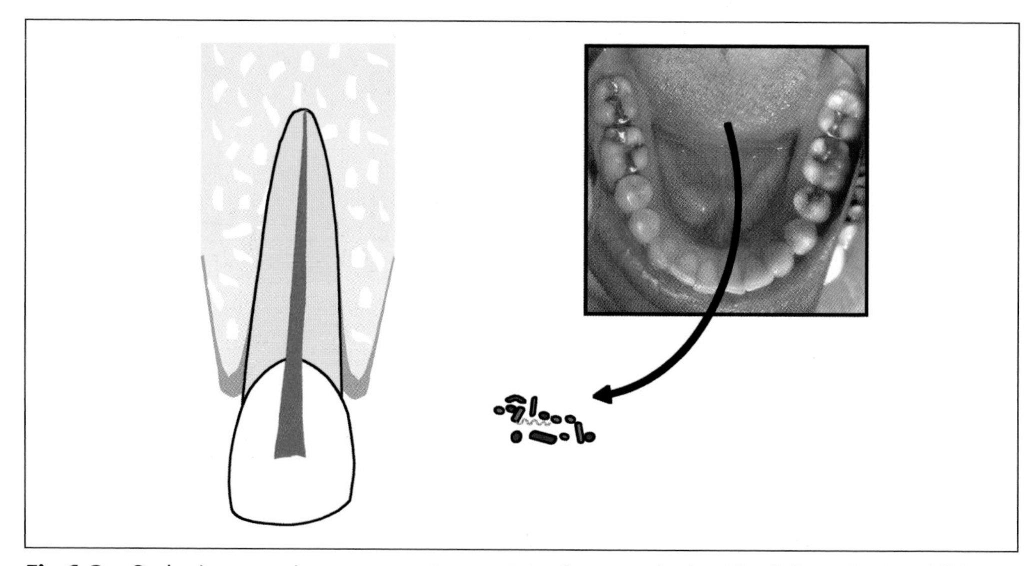

Fig 1-3a Oral microorganisms represent a constant threat to the health of the pulp. In addition to the immune response of the vital pulp, the enamel and dentin serve as physical barriers against their invasion, thus preventing apical periodontitis.

In apical periodontitis, a majority of the pulp space must be infected (Figs 1-3a to 1-3c). And for such a well-established infection to be present in the root canal system, the pulp must be necrotic. **Therefore, from a clinical perspective, a tooth with apical periodontitis of endodontic origin will test nonvital to sensitivity tests!**

If apical periodontitis is characterized by an infected and necrotic pulp, an obvious question is, What role does the vital pulp have in endodontic disease? If it is true that

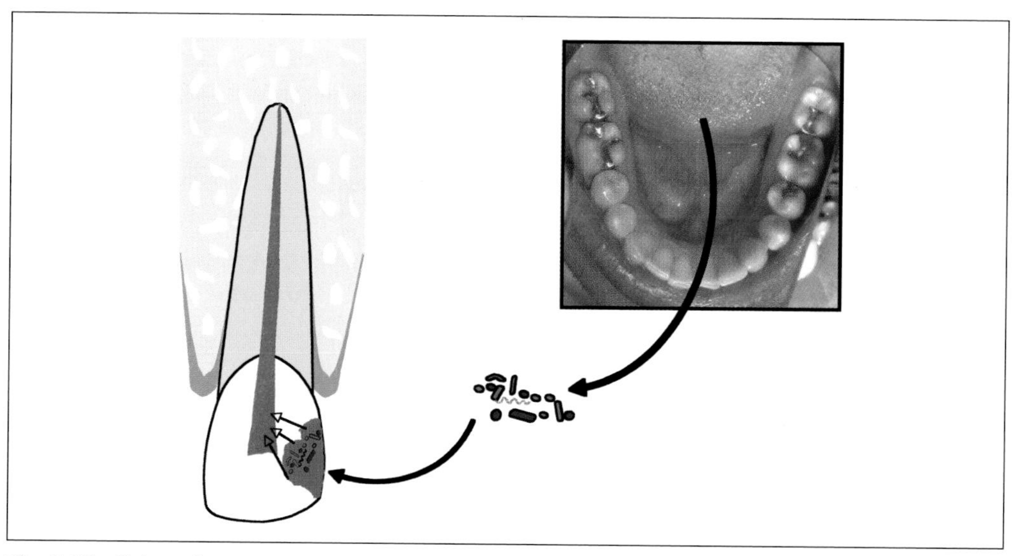

Fig 1-3b If the microorganisms are able to penetrate the enamel and dentin, the pulp will exhibit an inflammatory response (reversible or irreversible). If the pulp is directly exposed to the microorganisms, a zone of necrosis circumscribed by a zone of inflammation will develop. Over time, the necrotic zone will enlarge, pushing the circumscribed zone of inflammation toward the apex.

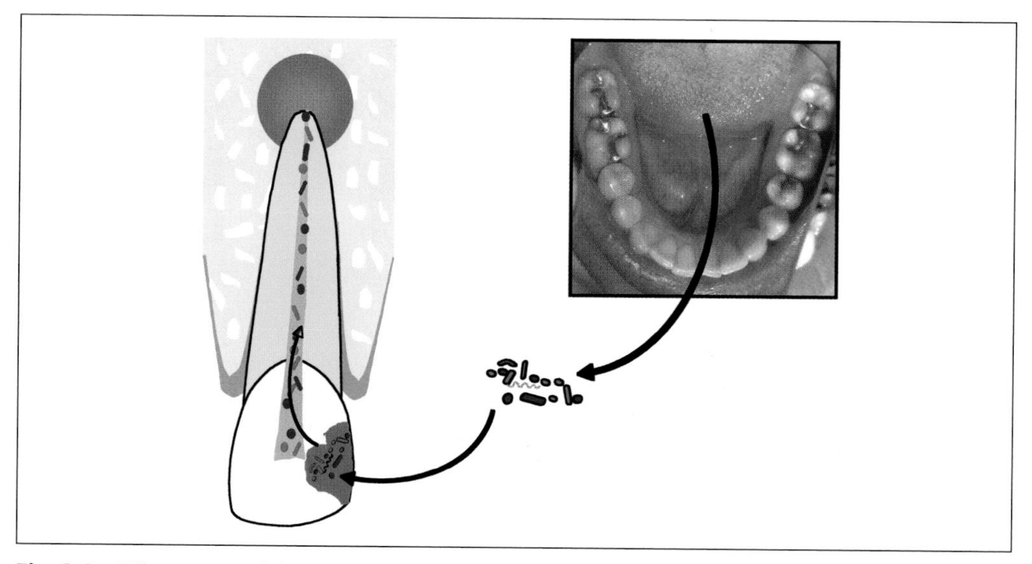

Fig 1-3c When most of the pulp is necrotic, the inflammation will move through the apical foramen, resulting in apical periodontitis.

necrosis and infection are essential components of the disease, it is also true that a pulp that is found to be "mostly" vital cannot be diagnosed as apical periodontitis of endodontic origin. **Therefore, maintenance of pulpal vitality or removal of the pulp while it is still vital will prevent the development of apical periodontitis.**

Thus, endodontics is the prevention or elimination of apical periodontitis. Prevention of apical periodontitis is achieved by vital pulp therapy, and elimination of apical periodontitis is achieved by a disinfection protocol of the root canal system.

As will be explained in a later chapter, a vital pulp cannot be considered as requiring the same treatment strategy as a necrotic infected pulp if one is to expect the same probability of success in both cases.

Vital Pulp Therapy

Vital pulp therapy can be divided into two categories: treatment of *reversible pulpitis* and treatment of *irreversible pulpitis*. These diagnostic terms imply that if a group of teeth with the history, signs, and symptoms of a reversible pulpitis were treated with standard operative procedures, most of the pulps would be expected to reverse to a healthy state. Since a healthy pulp cannot be associated with apical periodontitis of endodontic origin, treatment that will reverse an inflamed pulp to health is the best endodontic treatment that can be performed (Fig 1-4).

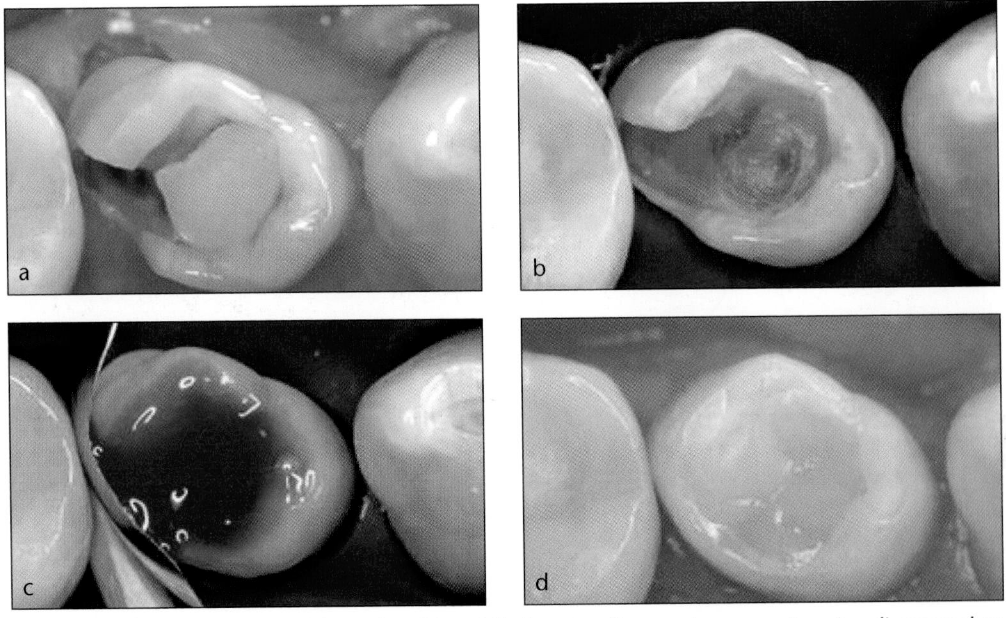

Fig 1-4 Vital pulp therapy. *(a)* Tooth with a failed restoration and recurrent caries diagnosed as reversibly inflamed; *(b)* Removal of caries; *(c)* Acid placement in preparation for a resin-bonded restoration; and *(d)* Final restoration. (Courtesy of Dr Andre Ritter.)

Conversely, if a group of teeth with a diagnostic presentation consistent with irreversible pulpitis were treated as above, then many of the pulps would become necrotic, infected, and develop apical periodontitis. Thus, the best preventive treatment in such cases would be aseptic removal of the entire pulp (pulpectomy) and filling of the root canal and coronal access (Figs 1-5 and 1-6).

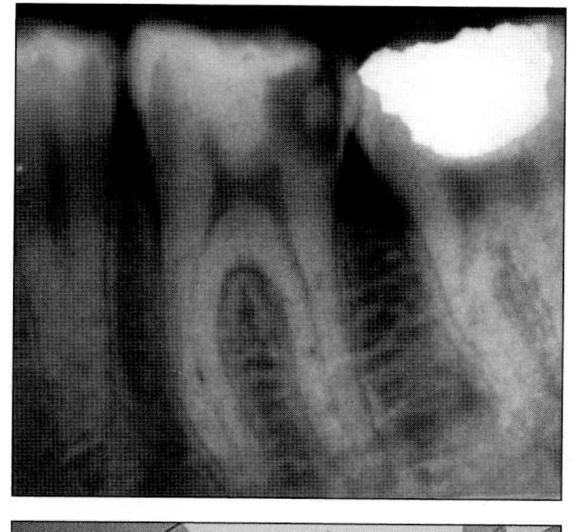

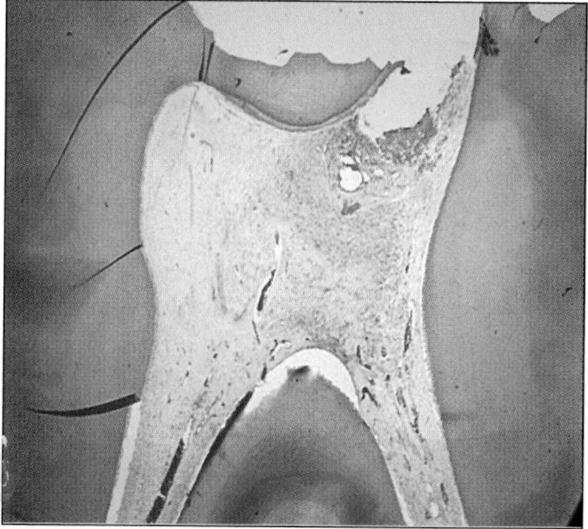

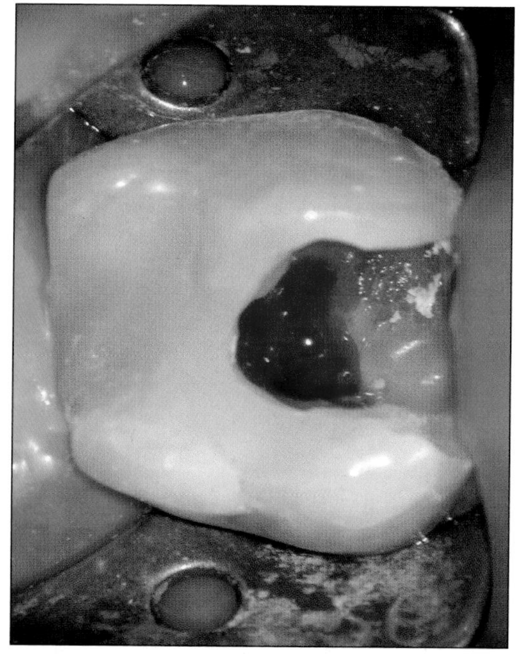

Fig 1-5 Tooth with exposed caries and symptoms of irreversible pulpitis (see Chapter 2). The most predictable treatment for the prevention of apical periodontitis is pulpectomy. (Courtesy of Dr Leif Tronstad.)

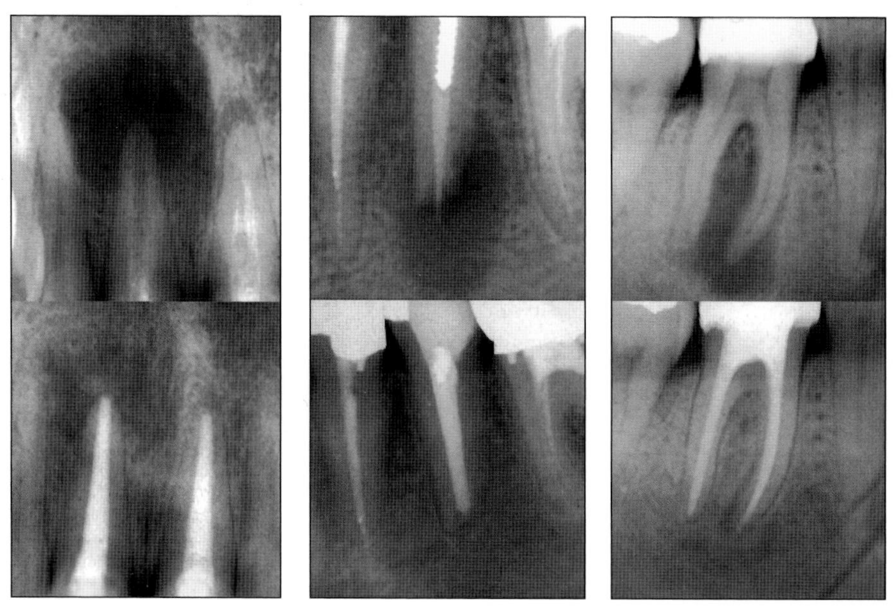

Fig 1-6 Pre- *(top)* and post-treatment *(bottom)* radiographs demonstrating healing in cases of distinct apical periodontitis.

Necrotic Pulp Therapy

Since microbes are the cause of apical periodontitis removal of the microbes should reverse the disease. A high probability of success in reversing apical periodontitis can be expected if the microbial count is lowered to negligible levels and the entire cavity (root canal and access cavity) is quickly and adequately filled and sealed.

Suggested Reading

1. Cohen R, Burns RC, eds. Pathways of the Pulp, 8th ed. St Louis: Mosby, 2002.
2. Mjör IA. Pulp-Dentin Biology in Restorative Dentistry. Carol Stream: Quintessence, 2002:39–76.
3. Ørstavik D, Pitt Ford TR. Essential Endodontology: Prevention and Treatment of Apical Periodontitis. Oxford: Blackwell-Munksgaard, 1998.
4. Tronstad L. Clinical Endodontics, 2nd ed. Stuttgart: Thieme, 2003:1–64.

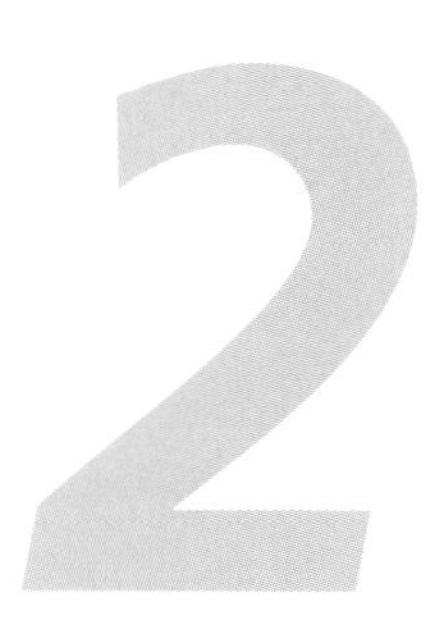

Diagnosis of Reversible Pulpitis, Irreversible Pulpitis, and Necrotic Pulp

As described in Chapter 1, different treatment approaches are needed for teeth diagnosed with reversible pulpitis, irreversible pulpitis, and necrotic pulp. Therefore, it is important to be able to recognize the diagnostic features that differentiate these three diagnostic categories.

While the type of pain experienced by the patient is often the factor that differentiates one diagnostic category from another, it should be emphasized that pain is the exception in both pulpitis and apical periodontitis (Fig 2-1). Therefore, clinical findings and knowledge of the reaction pattern of the pulp are essential in making a correct diagnosis.

It should also be acknowledged that the diagnostic tools presently used in dentistry are very primitive and rather inaccurate. For this reason, it is essential to gain as much information as possible from a number of different tests rather than to rely on one

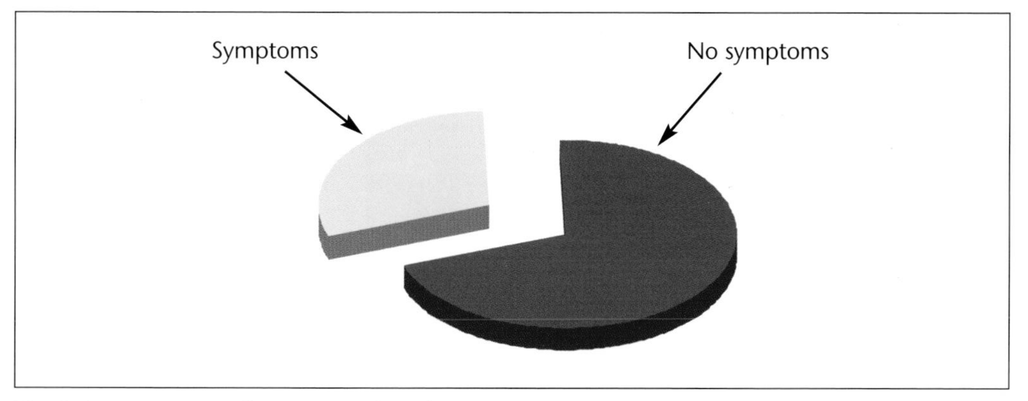

Fig 2-1 Proportions of patients with and without symptoms in cases of pulpitis and periodontitis.

particular favorite test. Ultimately, the practitioner must make as educated a guess as possible. But even the most careful and skilled practitioners can make incorrect diagnoses. For this reason, it is essential to follow up your patients and recheck the diagnosis. **Lack of pain is not the ultimate sign of success and in many cases is only temporary!**

The diagnosis is made after careful analysis of symptomatology, diagnostic tests, and the clinical exam.

Symptomatology

Chief complaint

The patient should be asked to state what brought him or her to your office. This could provide important clues about the status of the pulp and whether it is vital or necrotic, reversible or irreversible (Fig 2-2).

Symptoms Associated with

Reversible Pulpitis	vs	Irreversible Pulpitis
Pain-free		Pain-free
Sharp pain		Deep dull throbbing pain
		Pain to cold and hot liquids
		Pain to heat, relieved by cold
		Pain on biting

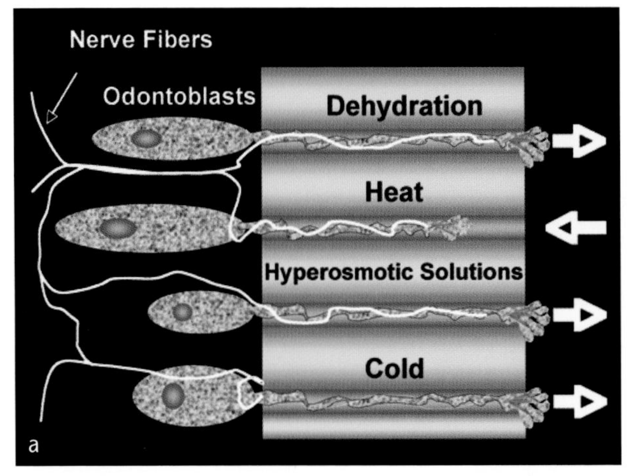

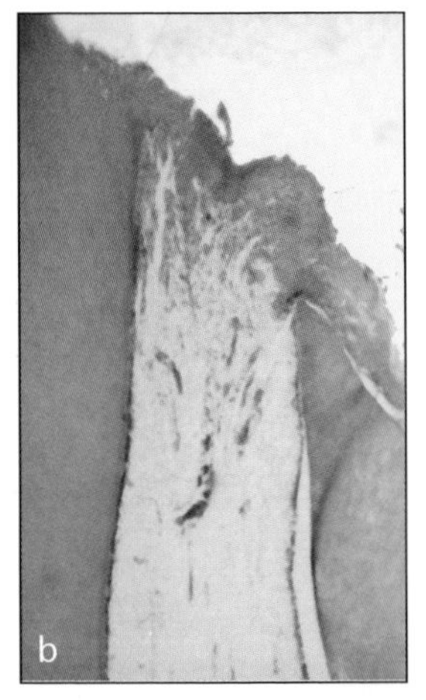

Fig 2-2 Reversible and irreversible pulpitis differ primarily in the nature of the pain each one causes. *(a)* Peripheral A-δ fibers cause sharp pain on stimulation. *(b)* Central C fibers cause severe, dull, throbbing pain.

Vital pulp: (a) No complaint, or (b) pain on contact with cold or hot liquids or with salty or sugary substances.

Necrotic pulp: (a) No complaint, or (b) pain on biting, pressure, constant pain. No pain in response to temperature. Pain can be but is not necessarily severe. Note: When the presenting symptoms confirm both vital and necrotic pulp, a cracked cusp or tooth should be suspected.

Reversible pulpitis: No complaint, or pain (usually mild) on contact with cold or hot liquids or with salty or sugary substances. Pain is sharp and goes away when the cold, heat, salt, or sugar is removed. Pain is not considered severe.

Irreversible pulpitis: No complaint, or pain on contact with cold or (particularly) hot liquids or with salty or sugary substances. Pain is severe, exploding, deep, dull, gnawing, pulsating, gaseous.

Differentiating features

Reversible pulpitis: Mild to moderate pain. Pain is sharp.

Irreversible pulpitis: Severe pain. Pain is deep, dull, gnawing, exploding, gaseous.

History of the chief complaint: The clinician must fill in any gaps left out by patients in their description of why they sought treatment.

Necrotic pulp: Questions should be asked to confirm that the pain is not temperature related and is present on biting, pressure, etc.

Reversible vs irreversible pulpitis: To differentiate between reversible and irreversible pulpitis, the patient should be questioned until some critical differentiation are made.

Nature of the pain

A key differentiation between reversible and irreversible pulpitis is the nature of the pain (if present). Reversible pulpitis is more likely when the peripheral A-δ fibers are stimulated. Stimulation of these fibers results in sharp, knife-like pain. If the centrally located C fibers are stimulated, however, the pain will generally be described in terms of severe, deep, dull, gnawing, and lingering. The latter descriptions are indicative of irreversible pulpitis.

History of the pain

In reversible pulpitis, the patient will usually report having had no previous experience of pain from that particular tooth. If the patient reports a past history of pain from the same tooth and describes it as spontaneous unprovoked pain, pain that wakes the patient at night, or heat-sensitive pain that is relieved by cold liquids, a diagnosis of irreversible pulpitis can confidently be made. In addition, severe pain that is difficult to locate accurately (referred pain) is indicative of irreversible pulpitis.

At this stage, the clinician should have a very good idea of how to diagnose the tooth in question. The remainder of the diagnostic process is directed toward determining which tooth fits this diagnosis.

Diagnostic Tests

As noted earlier, the tests used to diagnose pulpitis or necrosis are subjective and rather primitive. As such, when testing a suspicious tooth, the results should always be compared with the results elicited from a tooth that is thought to be healthy. The tests should also be repeated a few times to ensure that the patient's response is consistent. Generally, diagnostic tests are able to differentiate only between a necrotic and a vital pulp. They are presently not sensitive enough to differentiate between a reversible and an irreversible pulpitis.

Thermal tests

Thermal tests rely on fluid flow in the dentinal tubules. When cold or heat is placed on a tooth, the fluid movement in the dentinal tubules will result in irritation of the peripheral pulp tissue, including the A-δ fibers. A sharp "pain" will result. If the pulp is severely inflamed, it is also likely that the expansion (heat stimulation) or possibly that the contraction (cold stimulation) of the pulp tissue may cause stimulation of the centrally placed C fiber as well.

Cold test

The cold test should be performed using either dichlorodifluoromethane (–40°C) or carbon dioxide snow (–70°C). These agents are far superior to ethyl chloride (–4°C) or an ice stick from the freezer, which tends to melt on contact with the tooth and spread the cold to other teeth. For anterior teeth, the cold should be placed on the incisal third, for posterior teeth on the incisal aspect of the mesiobuccal cusp. These areas approximate the pulp horns, where the nerve innervation of the pulp is most plentiful (Fig 2-3). Before retesting the same tooth, the pulp should be allowed time to recover.

A consistently negative response is 97% proof that the pulp is at least partially necrotic and therefore in need of endodontic treatment. A positive response indicates a vital tooth. Unless the response is definitely of C fiber origin (deep, dull, gnawing, exploding), a positive response to cold in itself is not a sufficient basis to determine whether the pulp is reversibly or irreversibly inflamed.

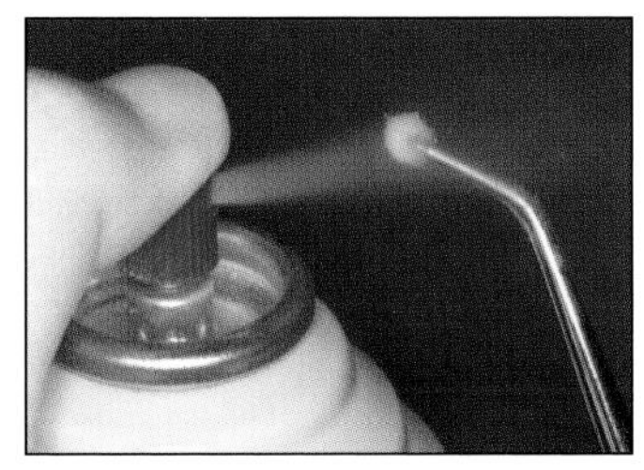

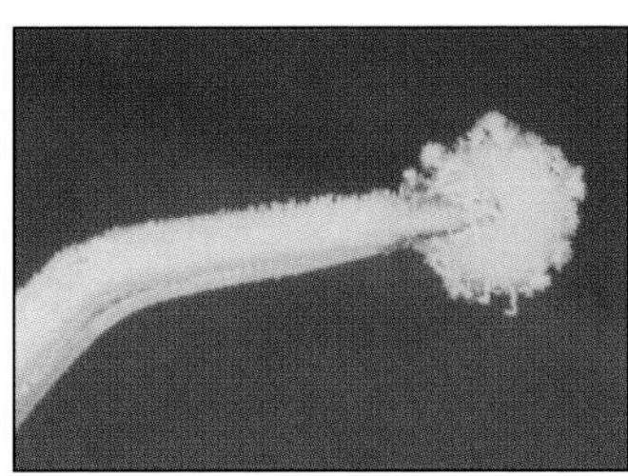

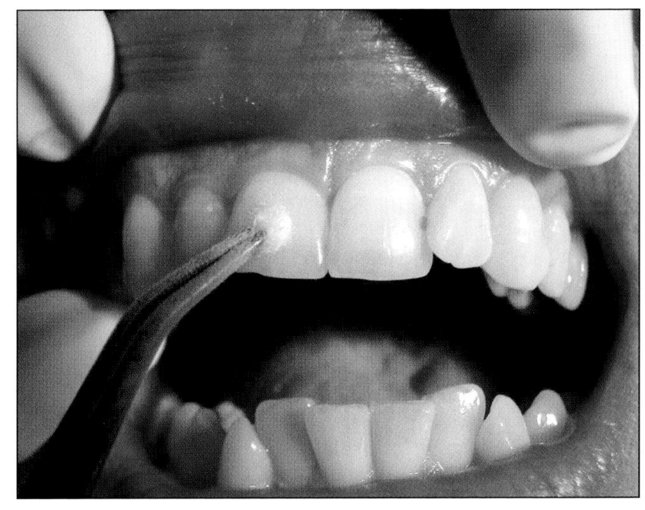

Fig 2-3 The most effective agents to use for the cold test are dichlorodifluoromethane (–40°C) *(shown here)* or carbon dioxide snow (–70°C), which should be placed in direct contact with the incisal third of the buccal surface of the tooth. The test can also be performed with an ice stick or ethyl chloride (–4°C).

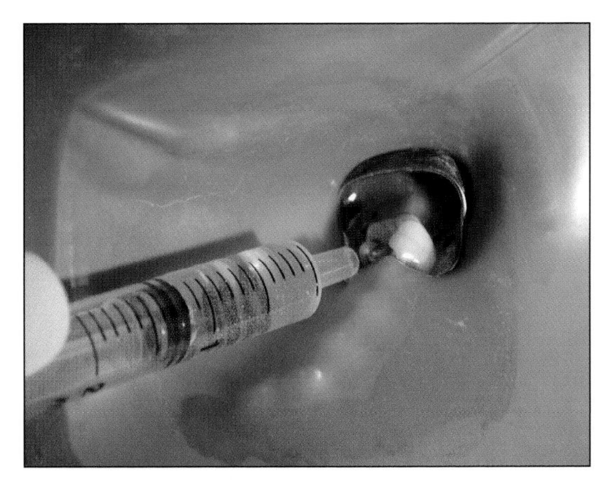

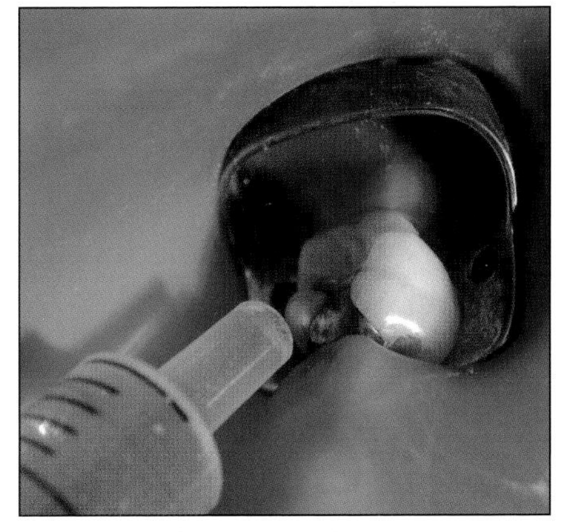

Fig 2-4 For the hot test, the tooth in question is isolated with a rubber dam, and hot water is gently squirted through a syringe until the entire tooth is covered. This protocol can be repeated several times using fresh hot water.

Hot test

At present, an effective hot test has not been devised. The best method of testing for heat sensitivity is to bathe the tooth in hot water. The first step is identifying the offending quadrant. Next, with the patient in a supine position, a rubber dam is placed on the most posterior tooth in the quadrant. A syringe is used to squirt hot water gently over the tooth until the entire tooth is covered (Fig 2-4). If this test does not reproduce the patient's symptoms, the rubber dam is repositioned on the tooth anterior to the tested tooth and the test is repeated using fresh hot water. This protocol is repeated until the pain is replicated. As with the cold test, a consistently negative response indicates a tooth that requires endodontic treatment. However, a positive response in itself cannot differentiate between reversible and irreversible pulpitis.

Electric pulp test

The electric pulp test (EPT) measures pulpal vitality through direct stimulation of the nerve fibers of the pulp. It is particularly effective in older teeth and in teeth that have limited fluid flow through the tubules due to dentinal sclerosis and obliteration. Again, the incisal third for an anterior tooth and the incisal third of the mesiobuccal cusp for a posterior tooth are the most effective areas for the EPT (Fig 2-5). As with both the hot and cold tests, a negative response is indicative of necrosis while a positive response merely indicates vitality.

Test cavity

When a previous restoration prevents thermal or electrical stimuli from passing through it, none of the diagnostic tests described here will be effective. In such cases, the only option is to drill a window into the restoration to allow the tests to be performed. Since drilling into the crown and dentin produces fluid flow in the tubules, this in itself, when performed without anesthesia, is an effective measure of pulpal vitality and is commonly referred to as a *test cavity*. In our opinion, test cavities should be performed only as a last resort and always in a situation that anticipates a normal or reversibly inflamed pulp. When performing a test cavity, copious water spray and feather touch drilling should be used.

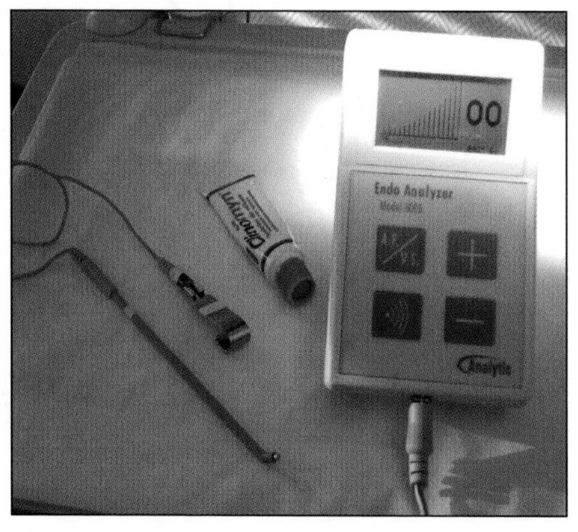

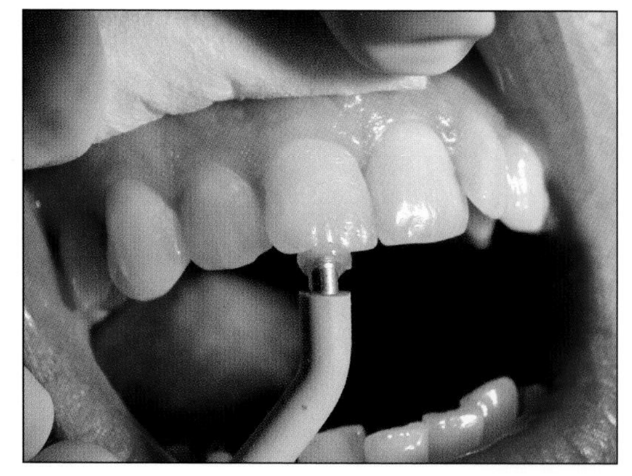

Fig 2-5 For the electric pulp test, an electrode is placed in contact with the incisal edge of the tooth to be tested. Toothpaste is used to ensure good contact.

Percussion and palpation

Percussion and palpation are used to evaluate the presence of periodontal inflammation. Since periodontal inflammation will be present in a necrotic pulp in the vast majority of cases, a positive percussion or palpation test is a useful additional indicator of apical periodontitis when the tooth has been nonresponsive to thermal tests or to EPT.

Also, it is possible that as it becomes necrotic, an irreversibly inflamed pulp can quickly lead to inflammation of the periodontal tissues, particularly through furcal canals or accessory canals that are high up on the root. If periodontal inflammation exists in a vital tooth, it is assumed that the root pulp is inflamed and thus reversibility of the pulpitis is unlikely. Therefore, a positive (hypersensitive) percussion or palpation test in a vital tooth is indicative of irreversible pulpitis.

The percussion test should be performed so that as much of the root surface periodontal ligament is "irritated" as possible Using the back of a mirror or another metal instrument, tap the tooth along the long axis of the root, since in most cases the inflammation will be at the apex of the tooth (Fig 2-6). The tooth should also be tapped in as many directions as possible to cover as many root surfaces as possible. While a hypersensitive response to sensitivity testing means that inflammation is present in the periodontal ligament, a normal response does not mean that inflammation is not present since the area of inflammation may have been missed in the testing procedure.

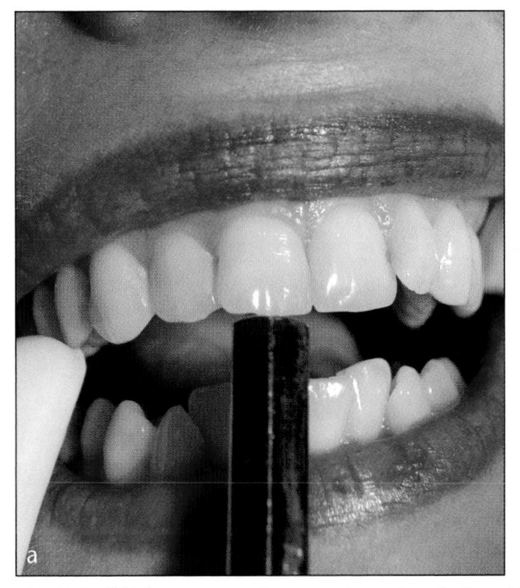

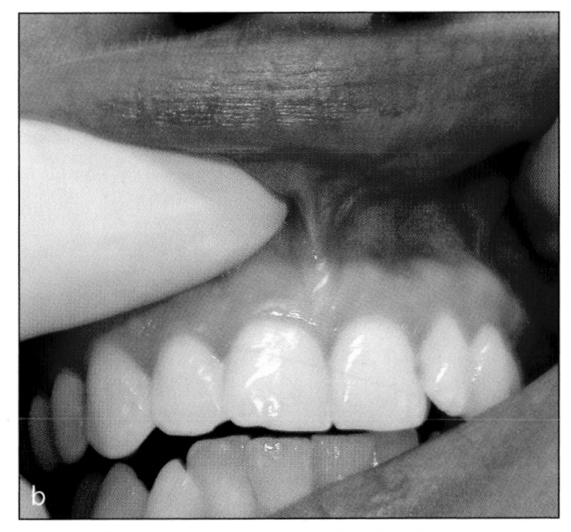

Fig 2-6 *(a)* The percussion test is a simple but highly useful examination method. The handle of a hand instrument is used to tap the teeth in a vertical direction. *(b)* The palpation test assesses tenderness, swelling, fluctuation, and crepitation in underlying tissues.

Palpation also tests for inflammation in the periodontal ligament; however, it is even more limited than the percussion test because it is only really feasible to test the facial surface of the apical part of the root (see Fig 2-6). For this reason, many areas of the root surface are missed by this test. It is likely that a positive palpation test is indicative of a necrotic infected pulp since only a fairly well-established periapical inflammation could cause pain on pressure through the apical facial cortical plate. However, in rare cases, it is possible to have a vital tooth with a hypersensitive palpation test that indicates irreversible pulpitis.

Radiographic Findings

It is not by chance that the radiographic findings are listed so low on the list of diagnostic tests. It is important to remember that a radiograph is a two-dimensional picture of grayscales and thus seriously limited in its diagnostic information. Too often, clinicians rely exclusively on the radiograph for the entire diagnosis!

A tooth with a necrotic pulp and apical periodontitis will probably, though not always, show a periapical/peri-radicular radiolucency. A tooth with reversible pulpitis will not show a periapical radiolucency. A tooth with irreversible pulpitis should not but may (rarely) show a periapical thickening of the lamina dura (Fig 2-7).

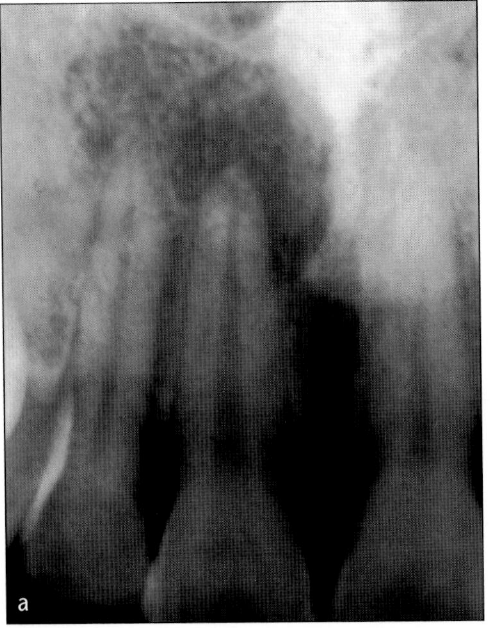

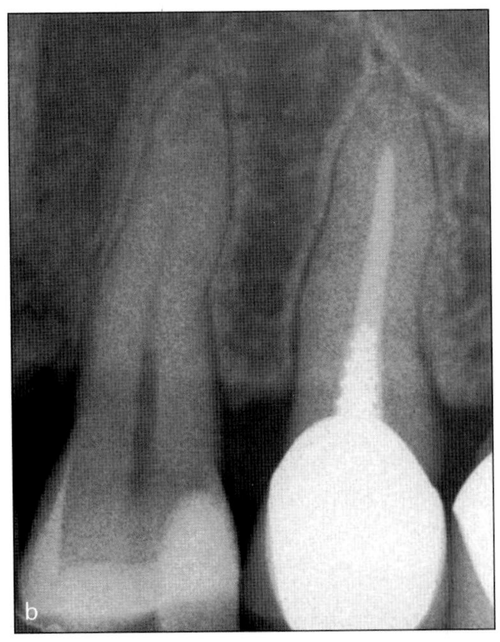

Fig 2-7 Typical radiographic appearance of *(a)* necrotic pulp with chronic apical periodontitis, and *(b)* vital and reversibly inflamed pulp.

Clinical Findings

After assessing the patient's symptoms and the findings of the diagnostic tests, the clinician should be able to reach a diagnosis and identify which tooth is the culprit. In most cases, the clinical findings will validate the diagnosis. Sometimes, however, the clinical findings may lead the clinician to change the diagnosis.

Caries exposure in a mature tooth

Currently, there is no vital treatment protocol that is consistently effective for the caries- exposed pulp in a mature tooth. Since the aim of treatment is to prevent apical periodontitis, in these cases the most predictable treatment method is pulpectomy under strict aseptic conditions. Therefore, even if symptomatology and diagnostic tests point to a reversibly inflamed pulp, when the clinical exam reveals a caries exposure, the diagnosis would be changed to irreversible pulpitis. Other clinical findings that may change a diagnosis to irreversible pulpitis include a tooth with severe periodontal involvement; an "old" calcified pulp; or a tooth with obvious previous insults.

Suggested Reading

1. Cohen R, Burns RC, eds. Pathways of the Pulp. 8th ed. St Louis: Mosby, 2002.
2. Tronstad L. Clinical Endodontics. 2nd ed. Stuttgart: Thieme, 2003.
3. Trope M, Sigurdsson A. Clinical manifestations and diagnosis. In: Ørstavik D, Pitt Ford TR (eds). Essential Endodontology: Prevention and Treatment of Apical Periodontitis. Oxford: Blackwell-Munksgaard, 1998.

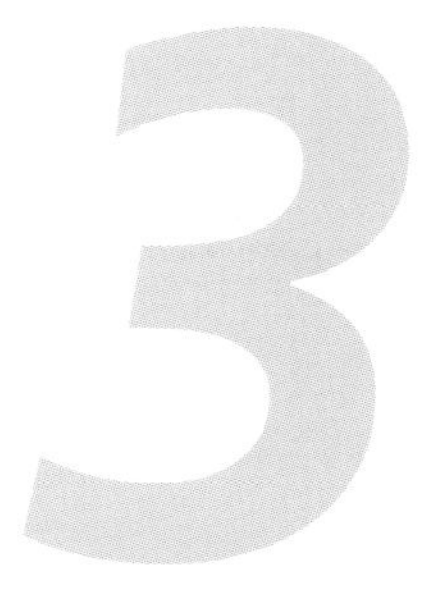

Root Canal Therapy: Defining and Achieving Success

General Principles

The previous two chapters introduced the different forms of endodontic therapy, including both *vital pulp therapy*, which involves superficial treatment of the pulp or treatment coronal to the root pulp, and *root canal therapy*, which involves treatment of the (vital or nonvital) root canal itself. The latter form of treatment, which applies only to those teeth in the diagnostic categories previously described as *irreversible pulpitis* or *necrotic pulp*, is the subject of this chapter. In certain cases, a tooth with a healthy pulp also may undergo root canal therapy because of restorative or other types of considerations.

Achieving Success

What constitutes success?

As noted earlier, apical periodontitis is the disease process of interest to the clinician performing endodontic therapy. Therefore, the absence of apical periodontitis subsequent to root canal therapy is the only true definition of success. Thus, for a vital tooth in which the aim of treatment was prevention of apical periodontitis, success is the maintenance of a disease-free apical periodontium. For a necrotic tooth in which apical periodontitis was clinically or radiographically evident, however, success is nothing short of eradication of the disease within a reasonable period of time (Fig 3-1).

It is important to emphasize that while time, profit, and postoperative pain are important short-term criteria upon which the patient and dentist may easily evaluate a treatment method, they cannot overshadow the most important long-term criterion for success—the absence of apical periodontitis.

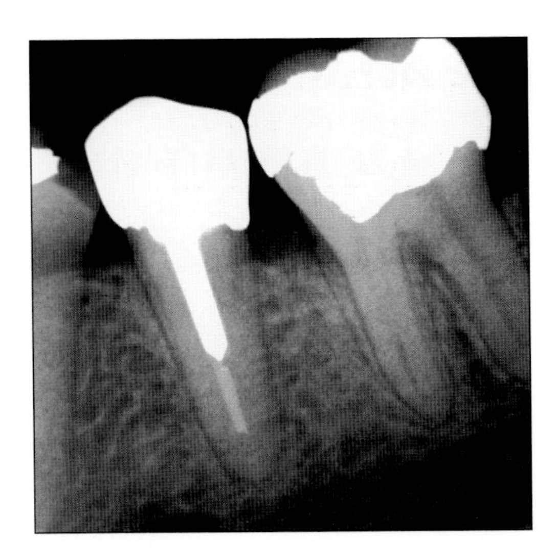

Fig 3-1a Successful endodontic treatment. Despite the poor quality of the root canal treatment on this tooth diagnosed with irreversible pulpitis, the 2-year postoperative radiograph confirms a successful result.

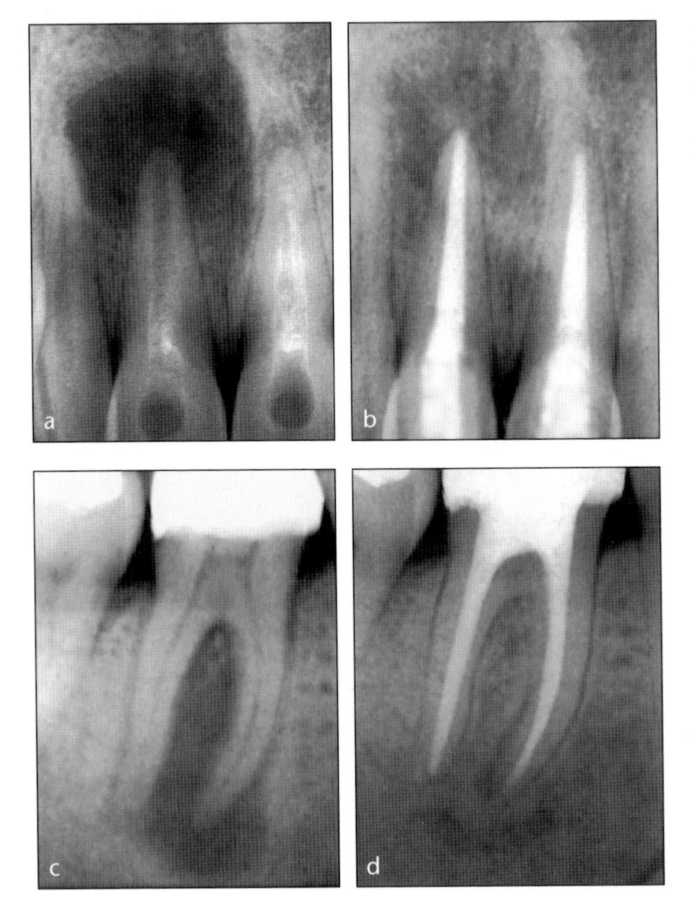

Fig 3-1b Healing is complete at the 2-year postoperative examination in these teeth with apical periodontitis (*a,c* preoperative; *b,d* postoperative).

Fig 3-2 Results of controlled outcome studies of roots with and without the presence of a radiolucency.

Bacteria and Prognosis

Success with vs without radiolucency

	No lucency	Lucency
Strindberg (1956)	89%	68%
Seltzer et al (1963)	92%	76%
Kerekes & Tornstad (1979)	94%	84%
Sjögren et al (1990)	96%	86%

Fig 3-3 Results of controlled outcome studies of canals that cultured negative (+) or positive (–) before root canal filling.

Bacteria and Prognosis

Success with (+) or (–) culture before root canal filling

	Culture (+)	Culture (–)
Engström et al (1964)	76%	89%
Zeldkow & Ingle (1963)	83%	93%
Oliet & Sorin (1969)	80%	91%
Byström et al (1987)		95%
Sjögren et al (1997)	68%	94%
Bender et al (1964)	No difference	

What are the requirements for success?

In nonvital teeth, apical periodontitis is caused by microbes in the root canal space; in vital teeth, where apical periodontitis is not expected to be found, the root canal is considered uninfected. Thus, it would appear logical that the absence of microbes in the root canal space subsequent to root canal therapy would ensure that apical periodontitis would heal (infected nonvital) or would not develop (vital)–assuming, of course, that the patient has a normal immune system. Controlled outcome studies appear to support this theory. When nonvital teeth that at one time were diagnosed with apical periodontitis and then underwent root canal therapy are compared to vital teeth, the vital teeth have a higher success rate—that is, a larger number demonstrate the absence of apical periodontitis (95% vs 80%) (Fig 3-2).

The explanation for the 15% lower success rate for nonvital teeth is that disinfection of these canals was not effective. Also, in studies where microbial cultures were taken of the root canals before they were filled, those that tested positive to microbial growth had a lower success rate than those that tested negative, which had a success rate consistently above 90% (Fig 3-3).

Of course, it is impossible to culture for all microbes that might be present in the root canal, and therefore many canals that tested negative for microbial growth did in fact contain some microbes. Nonetheless, the microbial threshold below which an extremely high success rate can be consistently achieved is well established and should be used to measure the effectiveness of any technique chosen by the clinician.

Summary

Fewer microbes in the canal at the time of root filling results in greater success. A treatment approach that results in a consistent (experimental) negative culture will result in success over 90% of the time.

Treatment Phases in Root Canal Therapy

Root canal therapy comprises two phases: the microbial control phase and the filling phase.

Microbial control phase

This phase of therapy is commonly described as *biomechanical cleaning, chemomechanical cleaning,* or *cleaning and shaping*. These terms all relate to the techniques with which the root canal is treated in order to minimize the number of microbes in the root canal space before it is filled. It is important to note that the technique used is not significant, providing that every means possible has been taken to establish a microbe-free canal before the filling phase is started. **Root canal filling should take place only when canal infection is controlled to the maximum degree possible.**

Therefore, the biologic aim of the first phase of root canal therapy is to clear the root canal space of all microbes. This should be accomplished without excessively weakening the root or affecting the tooth's capacity to be restored.

Teeth with vital pulps

Since the root canals of vital teeth are free of microbes at the start of treatment, the treatment principle for this category of teeth is theoretically simple—to ensure that the canal remains free of microbes at the end of treatment. Thus, the method of instrumentation is again not critical provided that adherence to a *strict aseptic technique* is maintained throughout the treatment. If an effective aseptic technique is used and the canal remains free of microbes at the end of instrumentation, it is logical that the prepared canal space and access cavity should be filled with a permanent restoration as soon as possible. Thus, if time allows for optimal attention to detail, both phases of treatment (microbial control and root canal filling) should be performed in a single visit. If possible, the coronal restoration should be placed during this visit as well.

If time is insufficient to complete the procedure in one visit, an intracanal medicament to prevent re-infection can be used in the same manner as for teeth with nonvital infected pulps (see below).

Teeth with nonvital pulps

Unlike teeth with vital pulps, teeth with nonvital pulps are almost always infected prior to the initiation of treatment. While an aseptic technique is an unwavering requirement for treatment of these teeth as well, a disinfection protocol aimed at the removal of existing canal microbes is required to achieve the aim of the infection control phase of treatment. Disinfection is accomplished via mechanical instrumentation, irrigation with antimicrobial solutions, use of intracanal medicaments between visits, and finally filling of the root canal itself to separate the remaining microbes from the surrounding periodontium, thus promoting healing (Fig 3-5). Even the most technically proficient endodontist is unlikely to consistently remove the optimal number of microbes from the canal through mechanical instrumentation and irrigation alone. Thus, to achieve the aim of the infection control phase of root canal therapy (minimal number of microbes possible), it is recommended that an intracanal medicament be placed into the canal for at least 1 week before the root canal is filled at a second visit.

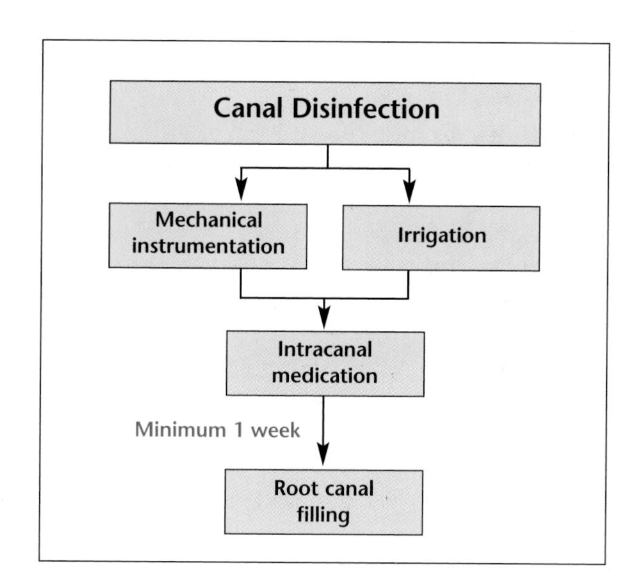

Fig 3-5 Principles of treatment for necrotic (infected) canals.

Stainless steel files and the step-back shape

The traditional technique for instrumenting the root canals of infected teeth is to use stainless steel files with a step-back shape. With this technique, a no. 25 file is used to the working length. This is followed by use of a no. 30 file that is 1 mm shorter than the no. 25 file and then by a no. 35 file that is 1 mm shorter than the no. 30 file. This process is continued at 1-mm increments until the length of the canal is treated from apex to orifice (Fig 3-6). After these "steps" have been created in the canal, a file is used to smooth them out, creating a conical-shaped canal with the narrowest part at the apical foramen, gradually increasing in diameter toward the canal orifice.

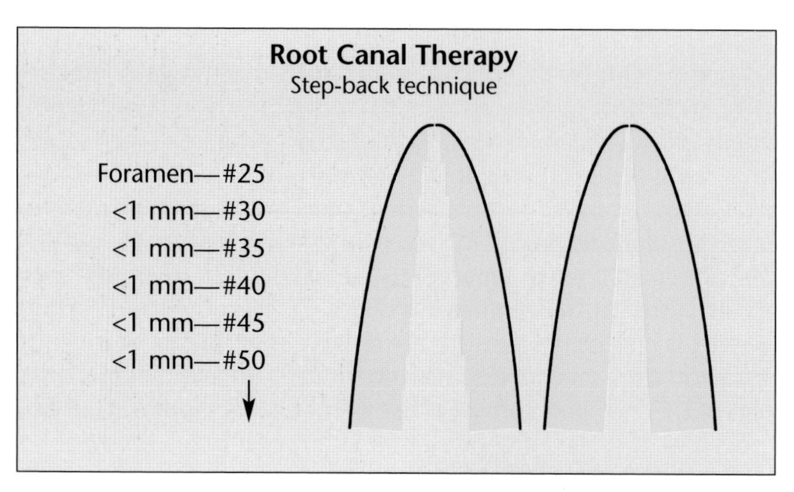

Fig 3-6 Step-back technique.

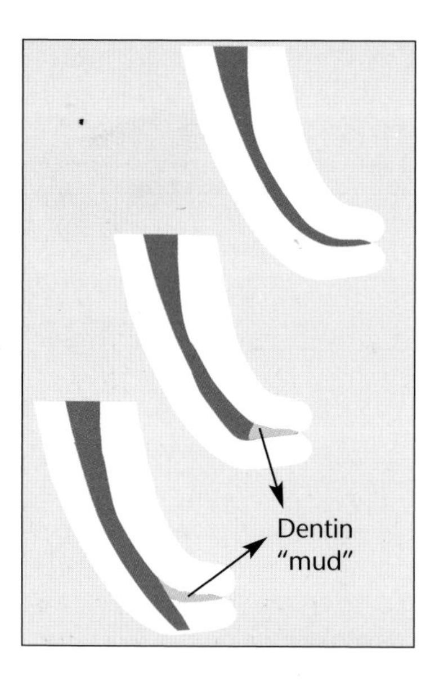

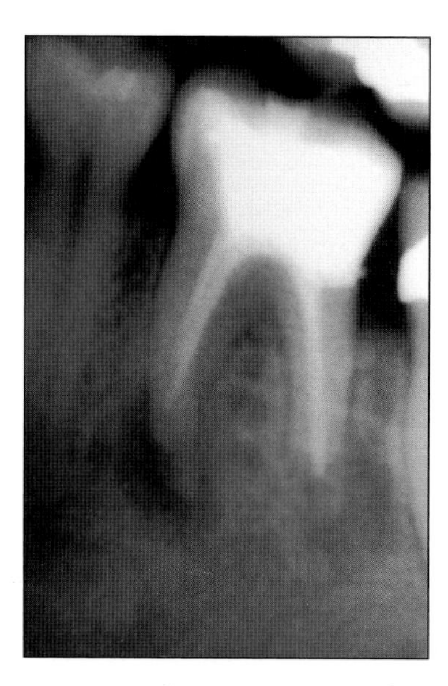

Fig 3-7 Effect of packing dentinal debris apically. The larger files are pushed away from the true canal, causing straightening or even perforation.

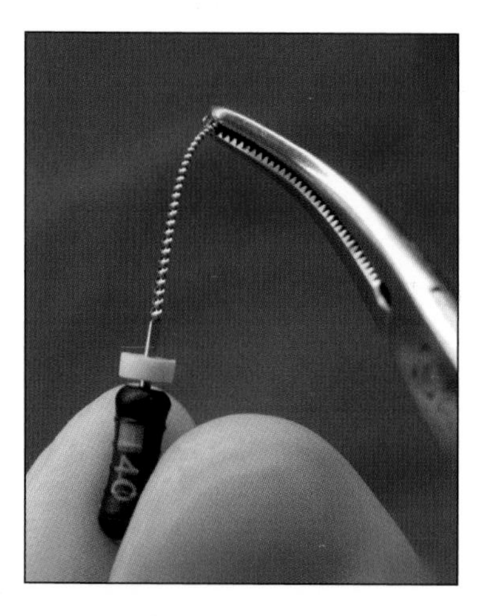

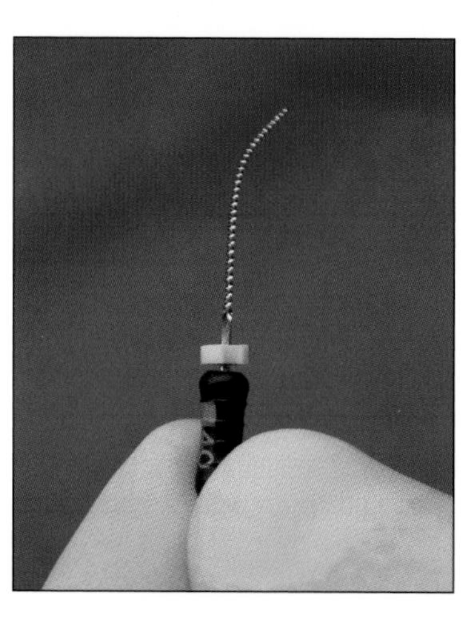

Fig 3-8 Stainless steel file no. 40 bent with a hemostat. The file is not flexible and therefore stays in its bent position.

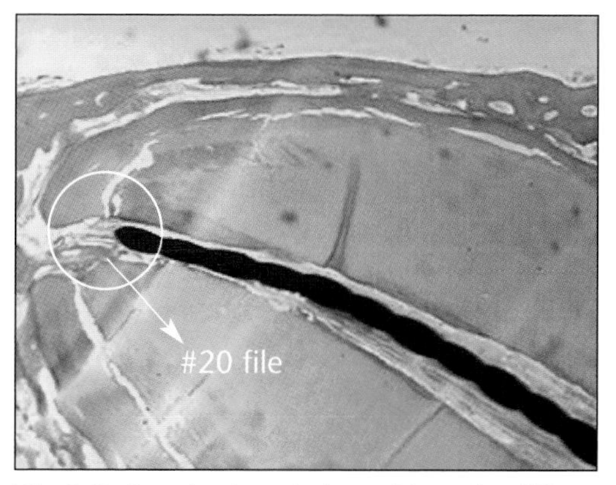

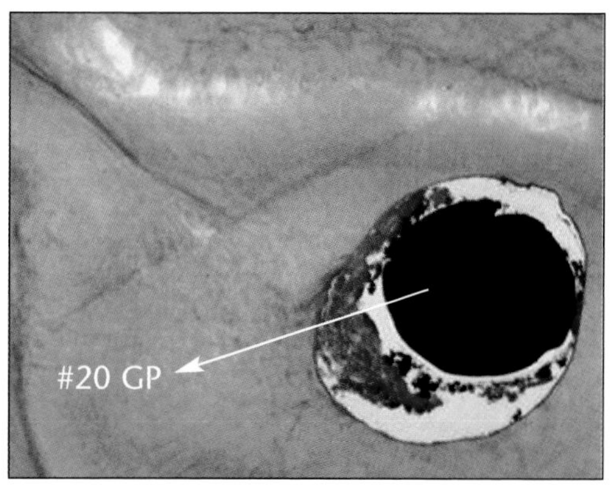

Fig 3-9 Step-back technique. Note the difference between the size of the true canal and that of a no. 20 file *(left)* or gutta-percha point *(right)*, even in the smallest canals. (Courtesy of Dr Richard Walton.)

While the step-back technique is safe in terms of procedural errors, it fails in the most critical aspect of the microbial control phase of endodontics: The size of the file at the apex is too small to adequately reduce the number of microbes to minimal levels. For this reason, the success rate for the treatment of teeth with infected canals is approximately 15% lower than that for vital uninfected canals (Fig 3-7).

Stainless steel files are precurved, but they become progressively less flexible as they become larger in size (Fig 3-8). This lack of flexibility in the larger files has been cited as the main cause of most incidents of apical blocking, straightening, creation of elbows, and strip perforations. In the authors' opinion, however, it is not the inflexibility of stainless steel files but rather the apex-to-crown approach to instrumentation that ultimately leads to most root canal failures. With this approach, as described below, a small file is maneuvered close to the apical foramen in an unprepared canal. The file now contacts the entire wall of the canal from apex to orifice. Instrumentation is initiated, producing a relatively large amount of dentinal debris throughout the length of the canal. In order to keep the canal unblocked and ready for the next larger instrument, all the dentin produced by the previous file must first be removed from the canal. In addition, this removal of dentin should be achieved coronally, not apically, in order to avoid blockage of the canal and the procedural problems already described. It is thus easy to see how instrumentation that begins with an ISO size 10 file and progresses to size no. 40 or no. 50 will lead to blockage of the apex with dentinal debris, causing shortening or straightening of the canal space (Fig 3-9). This is not the result of a lack of flexibility in the instrument, but rather the cumulative effect of using the 7th (no. 40) or 9th (no. 50) file in the sequence to remove all debris coronally. **The step-back shape is thus ineffective in achieving the biologic aim of the infection control phase of root canal therapy.**

Modified step-back shape

To overcome the limitations of the step-back shape of instrumentation, the modified step-back shape was devised. In this instrumentation technique, the step-back shape is accomplished first, since it is a relatively safe method of instrumentation in terms of procedural errors. After using a no. 25 file at the working length, the apical third of the canal is instrumented to larger sizes more appropriate for adequate cleaning of the canal (Fig 3-10). Thus, a size no. 30 is placed to working length and the sizes sequentially increased to larger apical third sizes. The use of larger–sized files is possi-

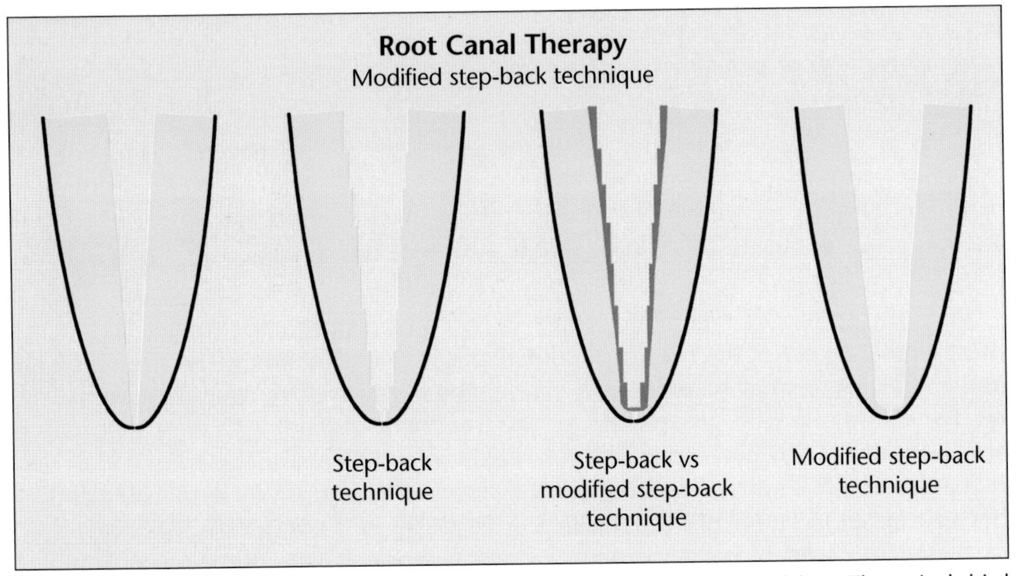

Fig 3-10 Modified step-back technique. The step-back shape is performed first. The apical third is then widened to biologically acceptable sizes.

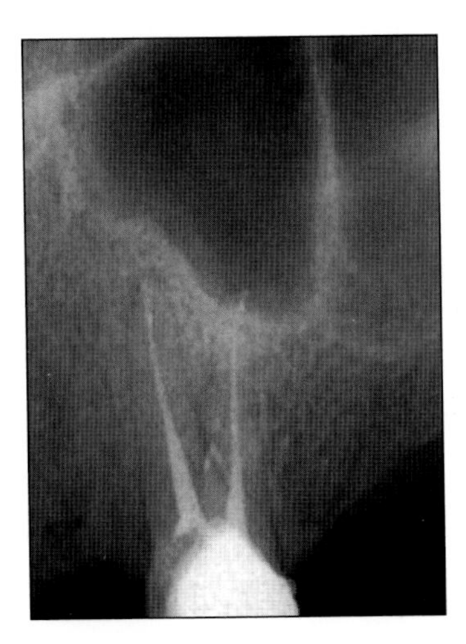

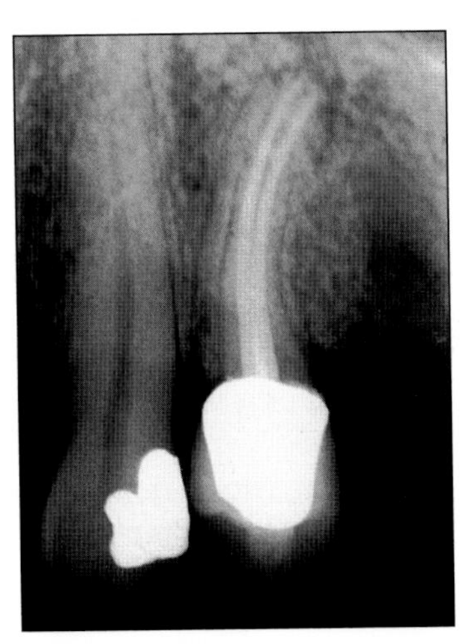

Fig 3-11 Radiographic appearance of teeth undergoing a step-back *(left)* versus a modified step-back technique *(right)*.

ble with this modified technique because of the space already created by the traditional step-back technique in the coronal two thirds of the canal. This space allows the larger files to be placed to working length, binding only the apical 3 or 4 mm of the canal. Thus, the dentinal debris produced by filing is much less than if the file contacted the entire canal, and there is adequate space for the produced dentin to easily move coronally (rather than apically). The modified step-back technique using stainless steel files will allow the practitioner to achieve acceptable microbial control in a more predictable fashion than the traditional step-back technique (Fig 3-11).

Crown-down technique with nickel titanium files

The past several years have witnessed a number of revolutionary changes in the instrumentation used for the microbial control phase of root canal therapy. The most significant change is the use of nickel titanium (NiTi) metal in endodontic files. NiTi files are extremely flexible and elastic. Moreover, they can be flexed under tension and then will "spring back" to their original size once the tension is released (Fig 3-12). Thus, they are easily able to follow curves in canals that were thought to be impossible with stainless steel files. The one disadvantage of this metal is its point of plasticity—that is, the point at which it stretches and the point at which it fractures are very close together. This means that if the metal is stressed, it can break without adequate warning to the clinician. However, if used carefully and according to instructions, fracture of these instruments is a rare occurrence.

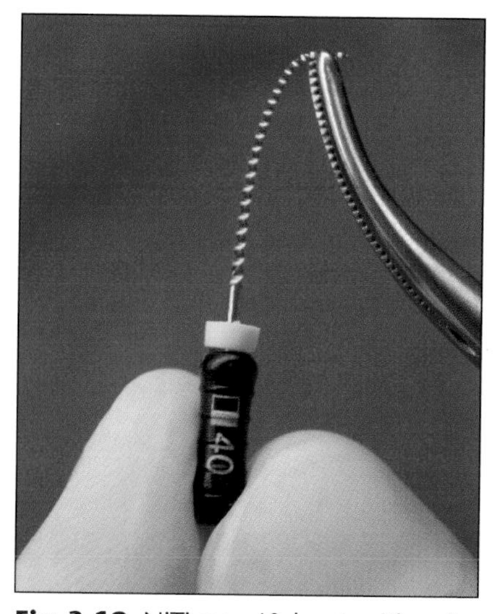

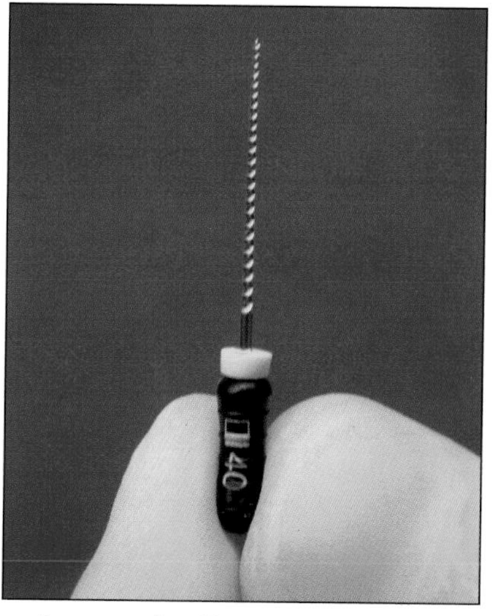

Fig 3-12 NiTi no. 40 bent with a hemostat. Because the file is highly flexible, it springs back to its original position.

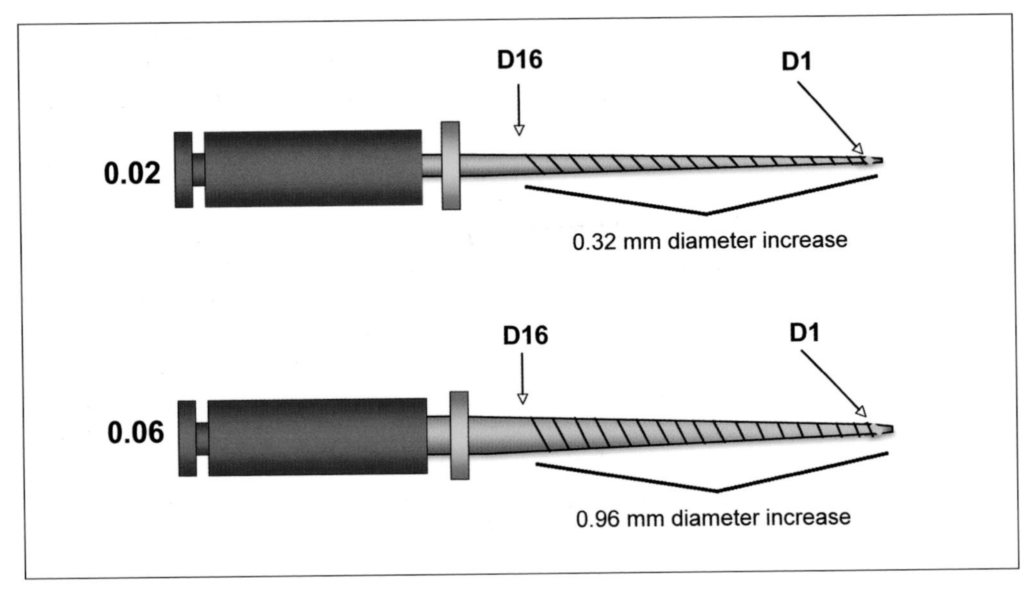

Fig 3-13 Variable tapers.

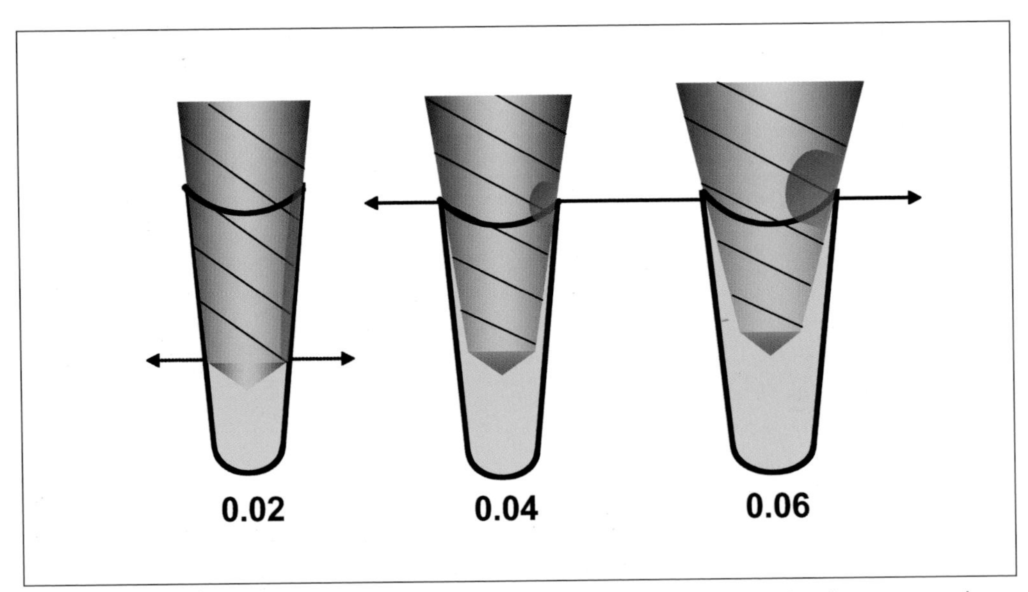

Fig 3-14 Effect of file taper on surface contact on the canal wall. Note that lower tapers leave less space apically and thus more debris can be forced in an apical direction, whereas higher tapers will cut more dentin coronal to the point of contact.

Another change in the file design within the last few years is the variability of the cutting length and taper of the files (Fig 3-13). Unlike stainless steel files—which were required to have a cutting edge of 16 mm independent of the overall length of the file and a taper increase of 0.02 mm/mm of cutting edge (0.32 mm total)—modern files have varying cutting edges and tapers ranging from 0.02 mm all the way to 1.2 mm/mm of cutting edge. A disadvantage of the larger tapered files is that the deeper they are placed in the canal, the more (unnecessary) coronal dentin is removed. A wedge shape is created, making the tooth more susceptible to fracture (Fig 3-14). It is therefore important to use the highly tapered files only in the coronal aspect of the canals and to decrease the taper as the file penetrates deeper into the canal.

As a result of the varying taper of the files, it is now possible to instrument root canals in a crown-to-apex direction, known as the *crown-down technique*, rather than in the step-back technique previously described. With the crown-down technique, a file is chosen with a taper that will allow it to loosely fit into the natural canal and then bind at the orifice, about 4 mm into the canal, when the taper becomes larger than that of the canal. When binding occurs, the file is rotated by hand or engine and the instrument moved apically in the canal. The file is advanced in 1-mm segments down the canal until the apical 3 to 4 mm of the instrument binds in the natural canal. At this point, instrumentation with this file should stop because too much of the file is binding, making breakage a distinct possibility and forcing dentinal debris apically. At this point, the next *smaller-sized* file, possibly with a smaller taper, is chosen to advance the file deeper into the canal. Because the smaller file is chosen, the requirement that the apical part of the file is loose in the canal is re-established and the file can safely proceed down the canal in 1-mm segments with little chance of breakage or blockout by dentinal debris. Thus, the working length can be achieved with relatively few files.

However, it cannot be stressed enough that while the working length at size no. 25 is much easier to achieve with NiTi files in a crown-down technique than with stainless steel files, at this point all that will have been achieved is the step-back shape, which we have already demonstrated to be inadequate for the microbial control phase of root canal therapy! Therefore, an additional step, similar to that required for the modified step-back shape, must be performed in the apical third of the canal. This step also is easier to perform with the new generation files. Indeed, sizes that are even larger than those obtainable using stainless steel files and the modified step-back shape can be safely achieved.

Summary

Nickel titanium files with variable tapers have revolutionized the way root canal therapy is performed. The initial phase of treatment is accomplished in a crown-to-apex direction, which creates space and allows for adequate cleaning of the apical part of the canal. The files are then used to adequately clean the apical third of the canal to sizes that will ensure the lowest possible microbial count before root canal filling.

Filling phase

The filling phase begins when the clinician is satisfied that the microbial count in the canal is at its lowest point. As stated earlier, this usually takes place during the first visit (time permitting) in the treatment of a vital tooth or following treatment using an intracanal medication in an infected necrotic tooth. The filling phase includes the root filling *and* the top or coronal filling. As its name implies, the aim of this phase is to fill the space created in the root and crown during the microbial control phase. If the space is optimally filled, remaining bacteria will not be able to communicate with the periradicular tissues, periapical exudates will not nourish remaining bacteria, and oral microorganisms will be prevented from repopulating the root space.

Suggested Reading

1. Cohen R, Burns RC. Pathways of the Pulp. 8th ed. St Louis: Mosby, 2001.
2. Pettiette MT, Metzger Z, Phillip SC, Trope M. Endodontic complications of root canal therapy performed by dental students with stainless steel K-files and nickel-titanium hand files. J Endod 1999; 25:230–234.
3. Schäfer E, Lan R. Comparison of cutting efficiency and instrumentation of curved canals with nickel-titanium and stainless steel instruments. J Endod 1999;25:427–430.
4. Tronstad L. Clinical Endodontics. 2nd ed. Stuttgart: Thieme, 2003.
5. Trope M, Sigurdsson A. Clinical manifestations and diagnosis. In: Ørstavik D, Pitt Ford TR (eds). Essential Endodontology: Prevention and Treatment of Apical Periodontitis. Oxford: Blackwell-Munksgaard, 1998.

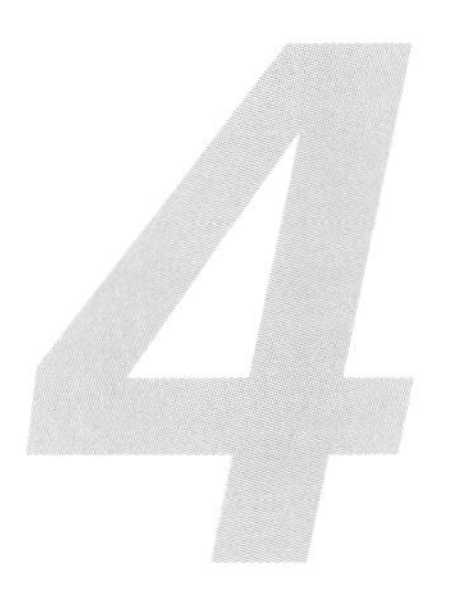

Root Canal Therapy: Clinical Procedure

Throughout this chapter, we assume that the tooth in question has been diagnosed and that it requires root canal therapy.

Estimated Working Length

It is essential for the clinician to establish an accurate estimate of the working length of the tooth before initiating treatment. This estimate is based on the preoperative radiograph, which should *always* be taken just prior to commencing treatment. In order for the radiograph to represent as accurately as possible the size and length of the tooth, the film must be positioned parallel to the tooth in question (Fig 4-1).

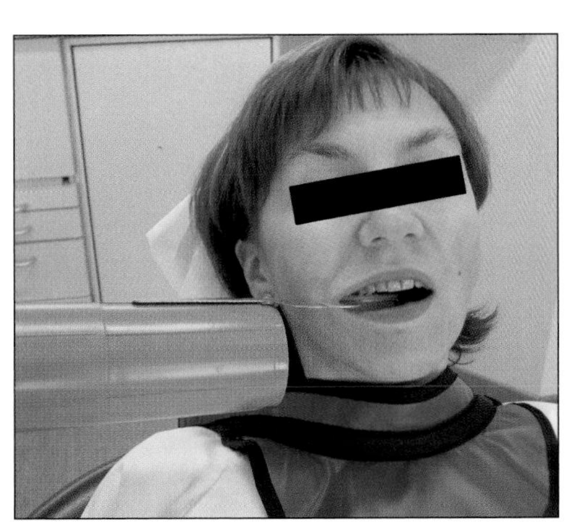

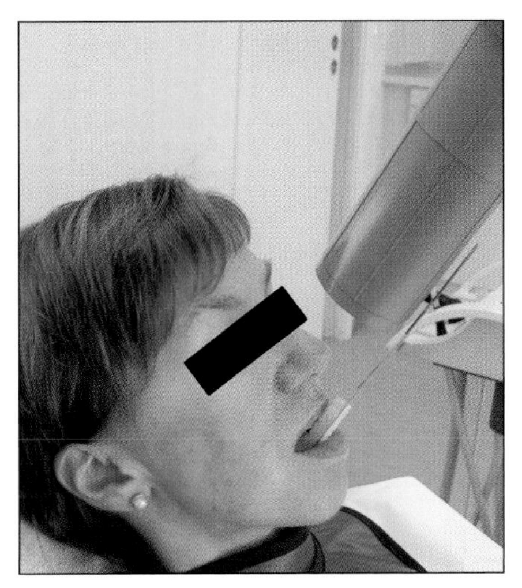

Fig 4-1 If placed correctly, the paralleling device will produce an image that fairly accurately represents the size and the length of the tooth.

A paralleling device will greatly simplify this task, especially in the maxilla; however, the clinician must bear in mind that this device ensures only that the tooth is parallel to the x-ray head and the x-ray film. The challenge for the clinician is to place the device so that the tooth is parallel *between* the head and film. In the mandible, it is much easier to ensure that the film is parallel to the tooth. However, the patient will need to lift the tongue while the film is positioned so that it can slip down parallel to the tooth (Fig 4-2).

The maxilla poses a much greater challenge. In many cases, the palate is too flat to allow the film to be positioned properly without causing it to bend and conform to the shape of the palate (Fig 4-3). Care should be taken to prevent this from occurring. Often the film must be placed toward the midline of the palate, and in these cases it is useful to place a spacer, such as a cotton roll, between the film and the tooth (Fig 4-4).

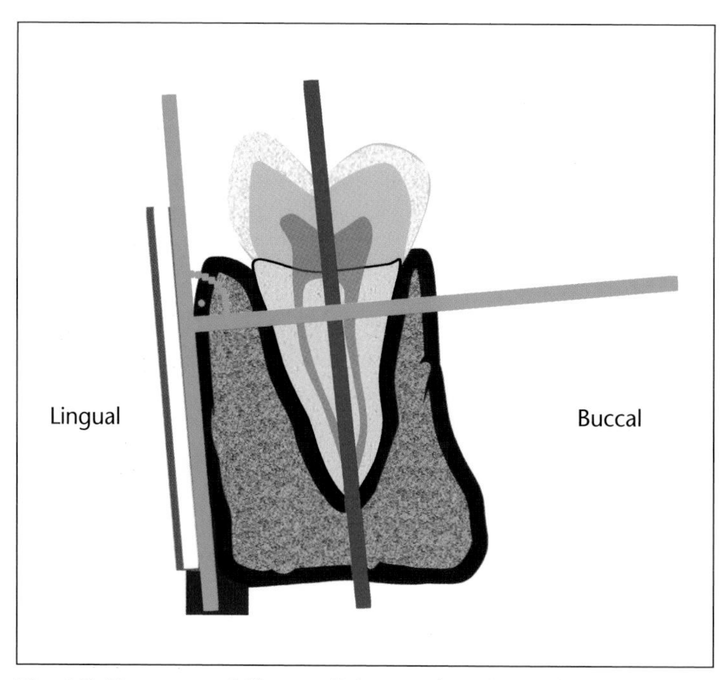

Fig 4-2 Placement of film parallel to tooth in the mandible. The parallel film-to-tooth orientation will produce a radiograph that accurately represents the length of the tooth.

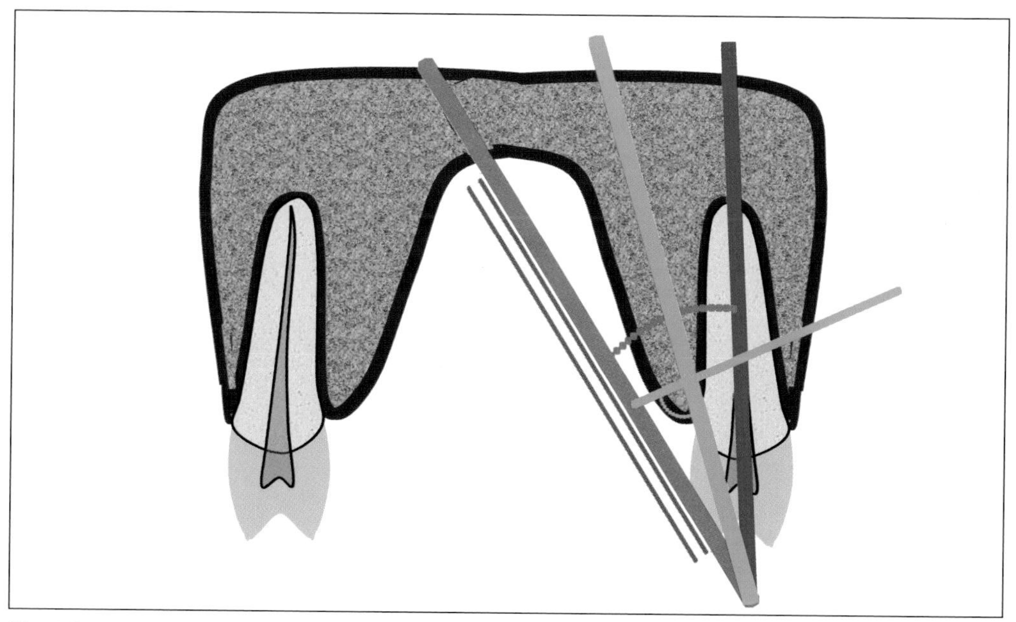

Fig 4-3 Bisecting angle technique with paralleling device. The shape of the palate makes placement of the film close to the maxillary tooth difficult. This difficulty must be taken into account when calculating the estimated working length on the radiograph.

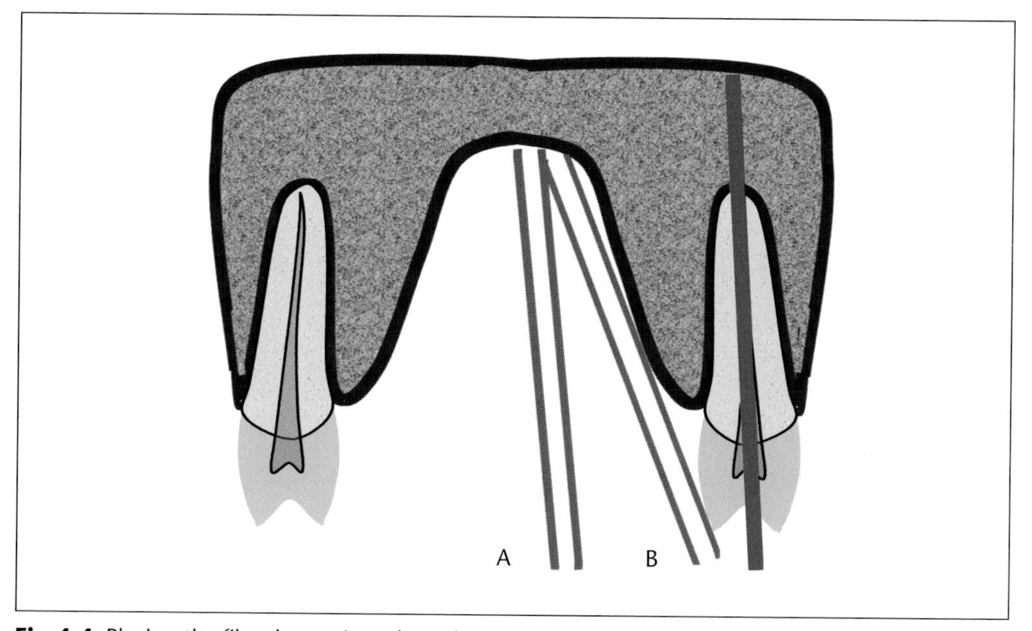

Fig 4-4 Placing the film deeper into the palate (A) will make it more parallel to the tooth. It is beneficial to place an object such as a cotton role between the film and the crown of the tooth to maintain its position while the radiograph is taken.

Once the parallel radiograph has been taken, a ruler or digital measuring device can be used to measure the tooth's radiographic image from its most coronal aspect to the apical tip of the root (Fig 4-5). Although this measurement is only an estimate—a fact the clinician should always remember—it will nonetheless allow the coronal two thirds of the root to be safely treated before the accurate working length is taken for instrumentation of the apical third.

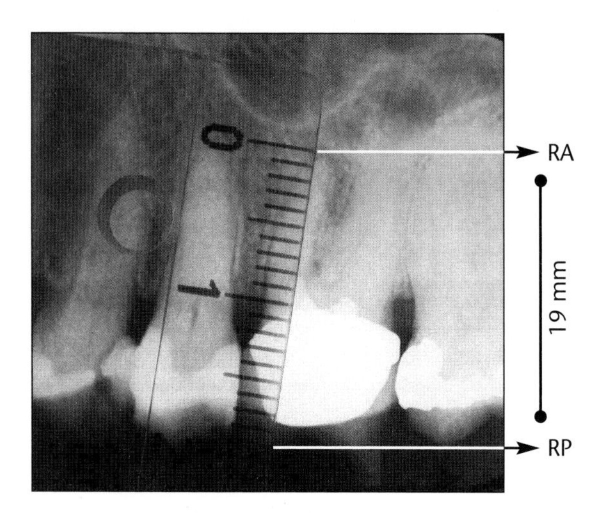

Fig 4-5a A ruler can be used to estimate the working length on a parallel preoperative radiograph (RA, radiographic apex; RP, reference point).

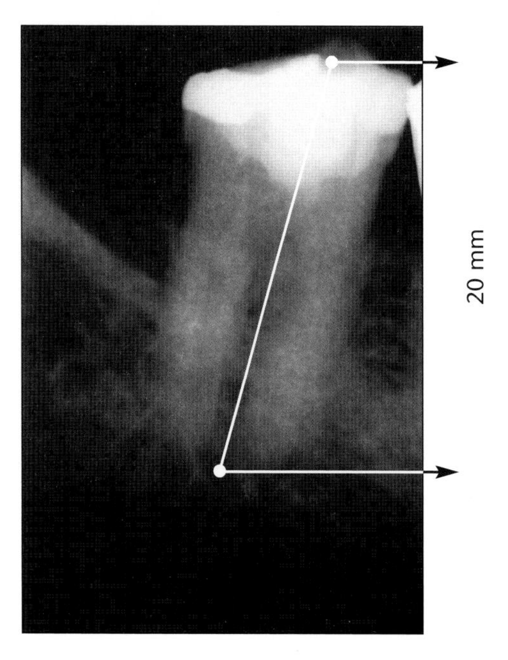

Fig 4-5b Measurement of the estimated working length on a parallel digital radiograph.

Access Cavities

Correct access is a key to successful root canal therapy. Straight line access cannot be compromised. With nickel titanium (NiTi) files, proper access is even more important because unlike stainless steel files, these files cannot be bent to facilitate entry into the orifice of the canal, nor can they easily be pushed against a particular wall of the canal for fear of breakage.

It is beyond the scope of this manual to review the anatomy and list the number of canals in each tooth. It should suffice to say that adequate treatment is impossible without a thorough knowledge of root anatomy (Fig 4-6). Remember that you will never find more canals than you are looking for.

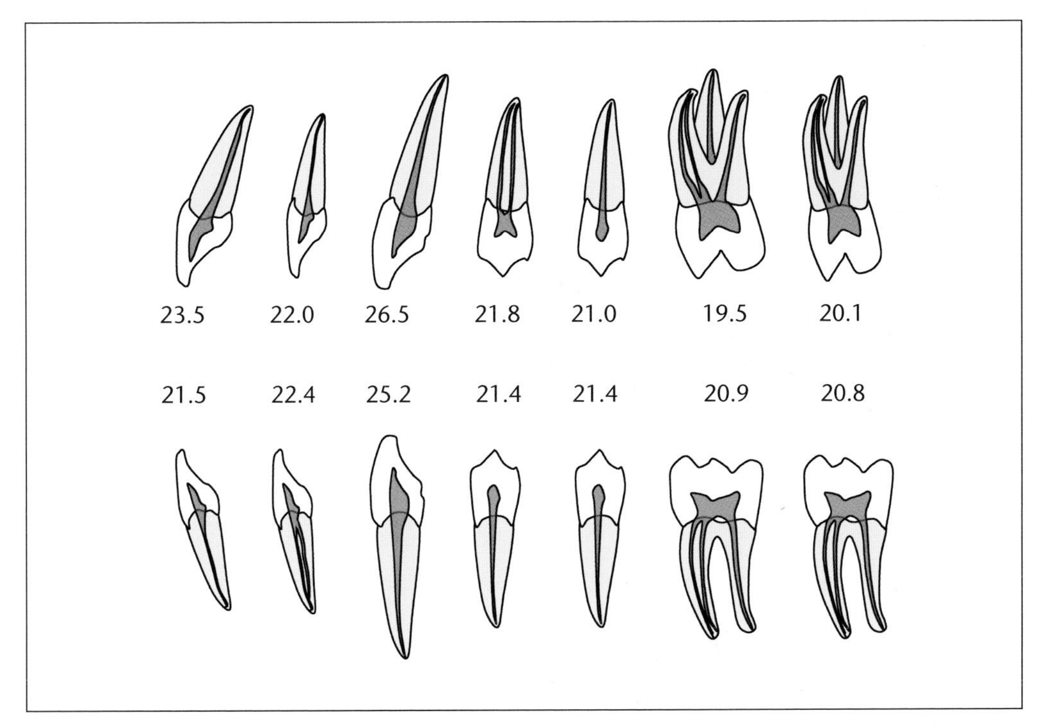

Fig 4-6a Average length (mm) of all teeth.

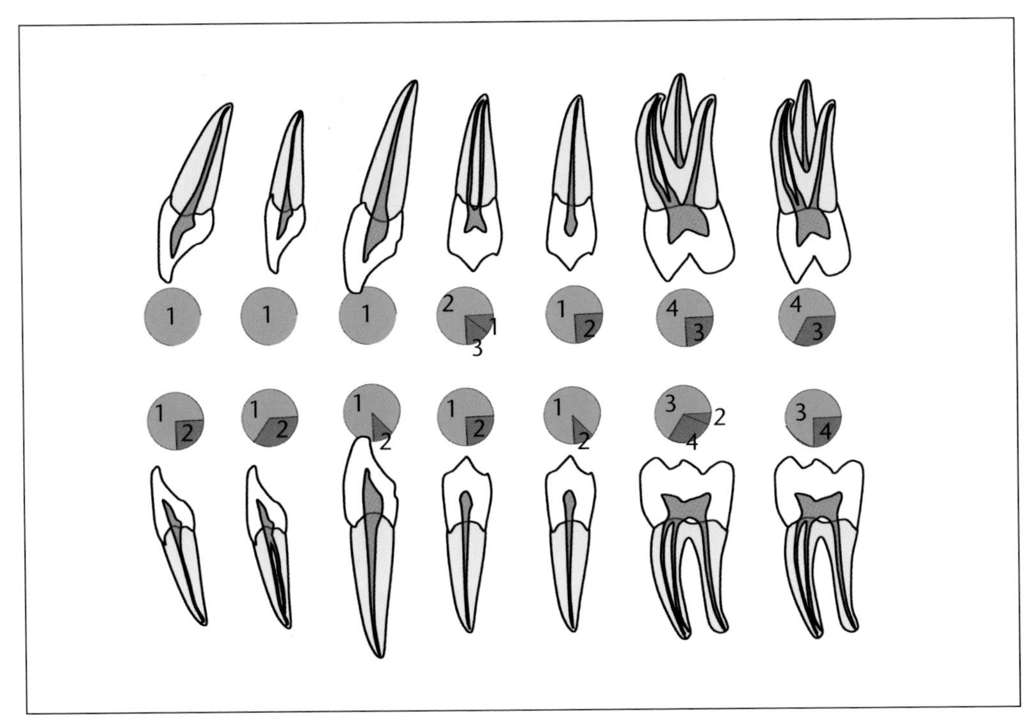

Fig 4-6b Number (frequency) of canals found in each tooth type.

Presented below are several tips to guide readers in creating access cavities that offer the best chance to adequately instrument the root canal.

1. The pulp chamber is always located at the center of the tooth; its outline is a miniature of the outer border of the tooth **at the level of the cementoenamel junction (CEJ)** (Fig 4-7).

   When starting the access cavity, the outer border of the tooth at the CEJ should be clearly within view; thus, if one aims for the middle of the CEJ, the pulp chamber should always be located. Once the roof of the chamber is penetrated, the entire roof can be removed by following the shape of the outer border of the tooth at the CEJ. From a practical point of view, the authors recommend making the access into the pulp chamber before the rubber dam is placed, since this will afford the best view of the CEJ. When the access is complete and all caries and leaky restorations have been removed, the rubber dam can be placed and steps can be taken to ensure an aseptic environment.

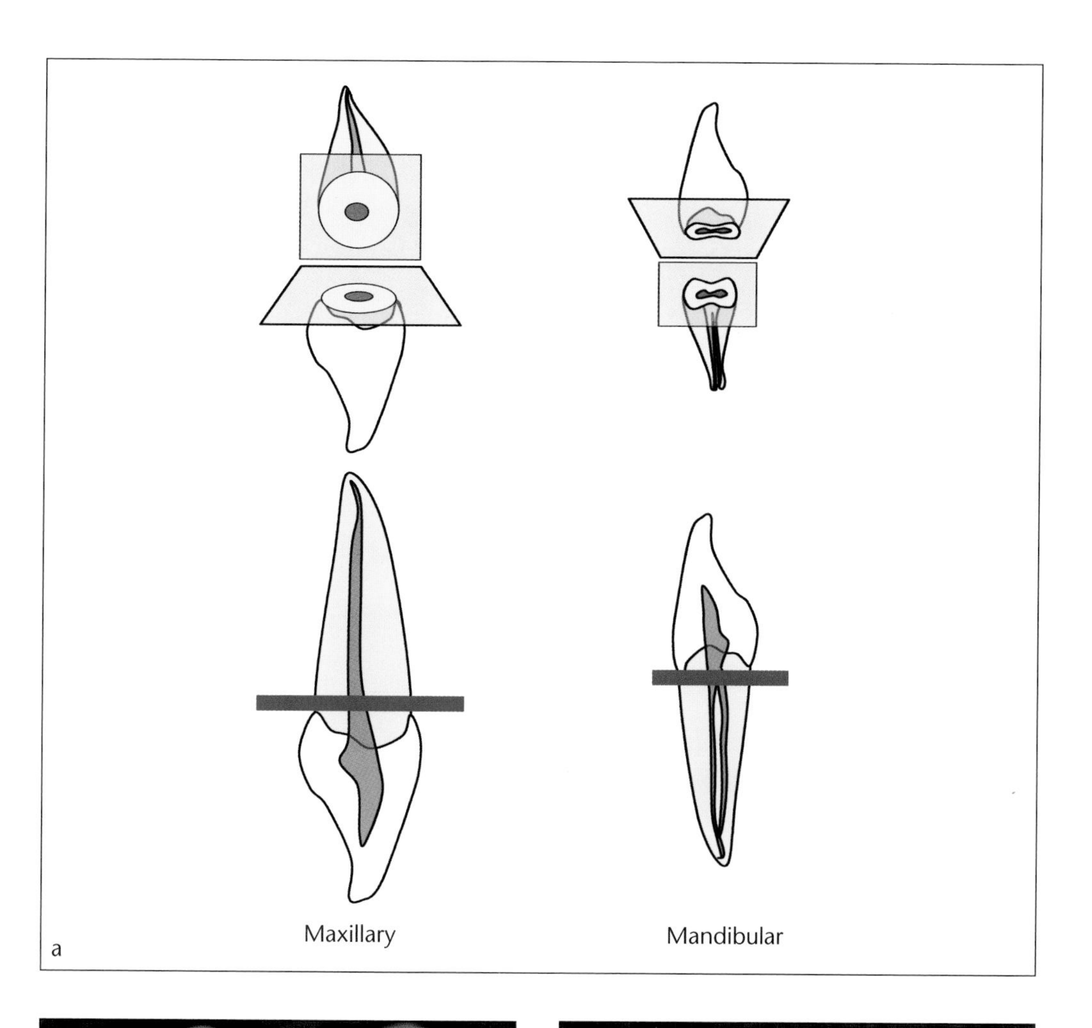

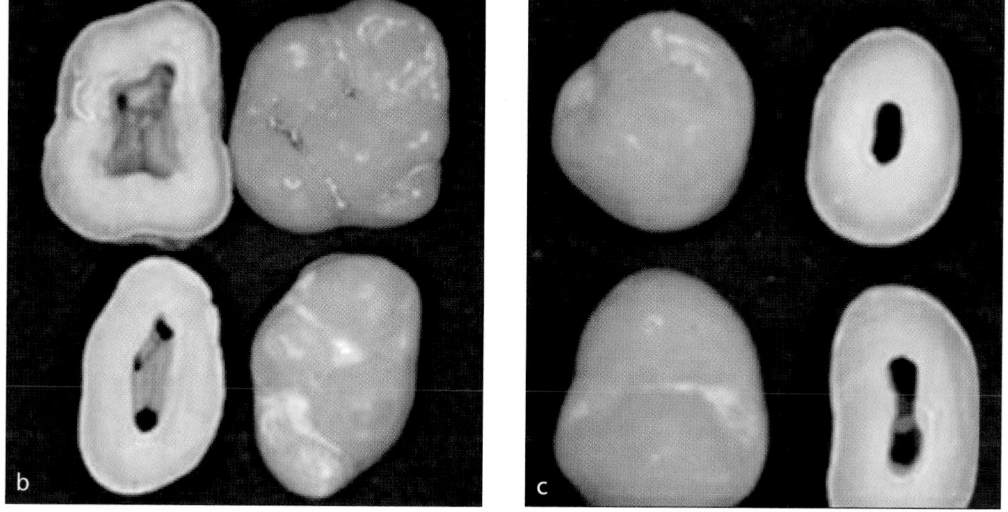

Fig 4-7 The shape of the pulp chamber mirrors the outline shape of the root at the level of the cementoenamel junction (CEJ).

2. The orifices of the canals are always located at the junction between the darker chamber floor and the lighter chamber walls and usually at the vertex of the dark-floor angle (Fig 4-8).

   Only when the junction between the dark floor and lighter wall can be easily distinguished is the access adequate. If this junction cannot be seen, it is an indication that the entire roof of the chamber has not been removed. In this case, the access must be enlarged by removal of the entire roof of the chamber. Once the access is adequately enlarged, it will be possible to use an endodontic explorer to probe for the canal orifices at the vertex of the chamber floor angles. The floor of the chamber should be drilled only when there is evidence that the canal orifices are calcified. In the vast majority of cases, it will be possible to find the orifices with an endodontic probe.
3. In teeth with multiple canals, the orifices are symmetrical to each other (Fig 4-9). If an orifice is found on one side of an imaginary line drawn mesiodistal through the floor of the chamber, one should expect to find another orifice equidistant on the opposite side of the line. If the orifice is located exactly on this line, it is likely to be the only orifice present, and it is not necessary to look for another.

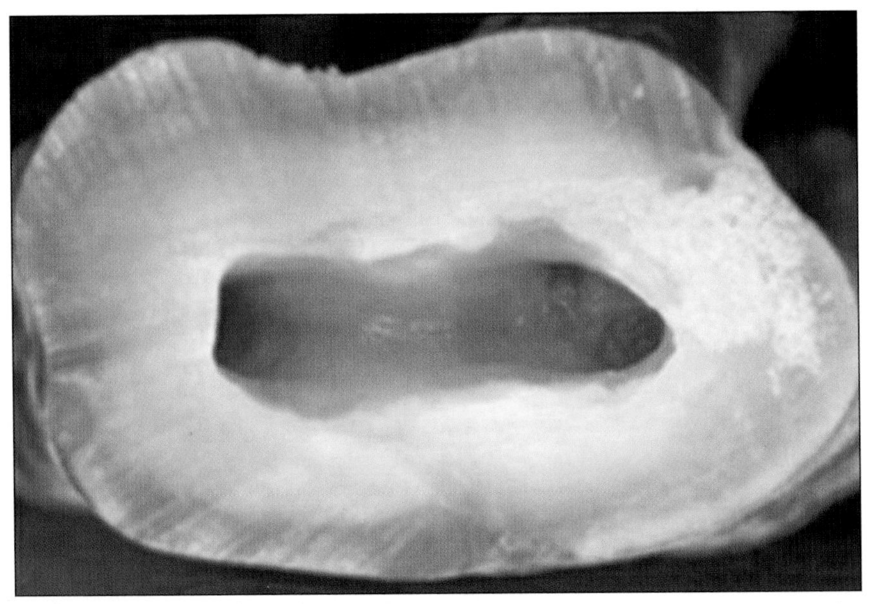

Fig 4-8 Occlusal view of an access cavity. The light walls meet the dark floor; the canal orifices are located at the angles of the dark floor. The access cavity is adequate when the junction between the dark floor and the light walls can be visualized.

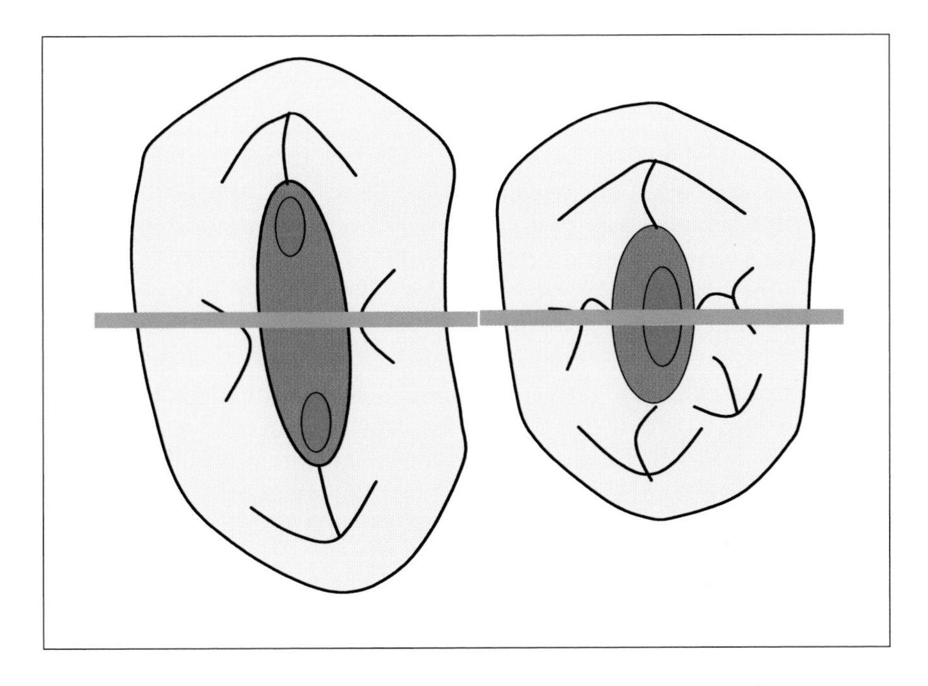

Fig 4-9 The canal orifices are symmetrical to each other.

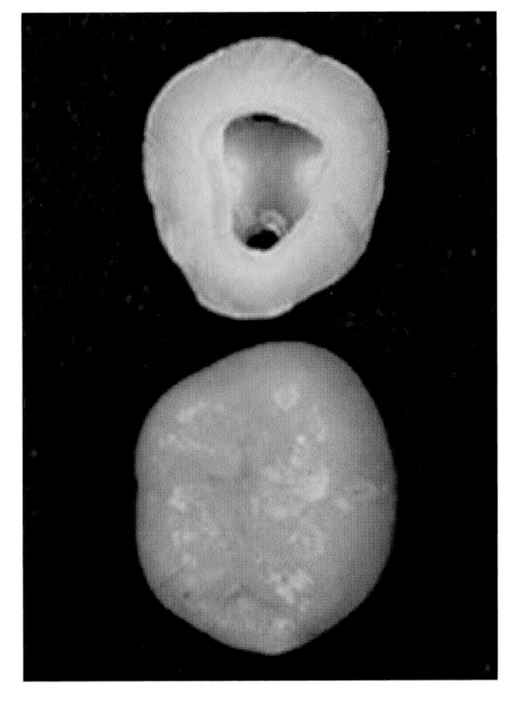

Aseptic Technique

Since the key to successful root canal treatment is controlling the microbial flora in the root canal before it is filled, it is critically important to apply a technique that does not result in contamination of the canal during treatment. Asepsis is the key!

While the importance of asepsis is simple enough to understand in theory, practicing strict asepsis is one of the most difficult tasks to learn, primarily because microbes are invisible to the naked eye. Some basic rules will help the practitioner and assistant develop a more effective aseptic technique:

1. Divide the treatment into "dirty" and "clean" stages. The dirty stage is performed before the rubber dam is placed and involves creating the access opening and removing ALL caries and suspect restorations. Do not compromise in performing these tasks. It is impossible to maintain an aseptic environment in the tooth if any caries remains. Moreover, if the tooth is nonrestorable, it is important to find this out before the root treatment begins (Fig 4-10).

   Once the caries and leaky restorations have been removed and the tooth is deemed restorable, the rubber dam is placed and the circumference sealed from saliva (Fig 4-11).

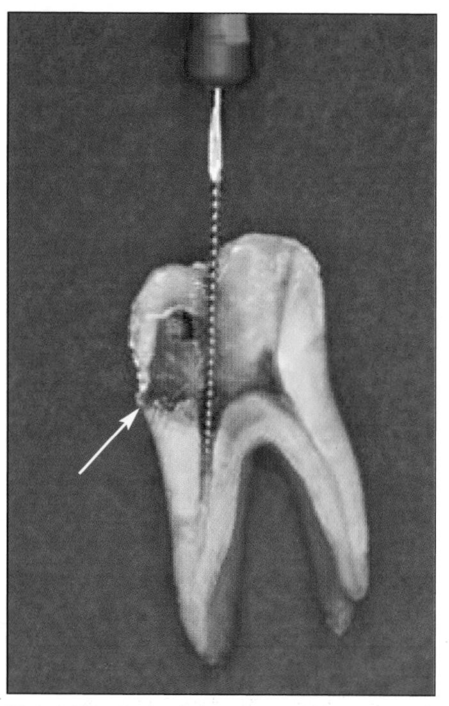

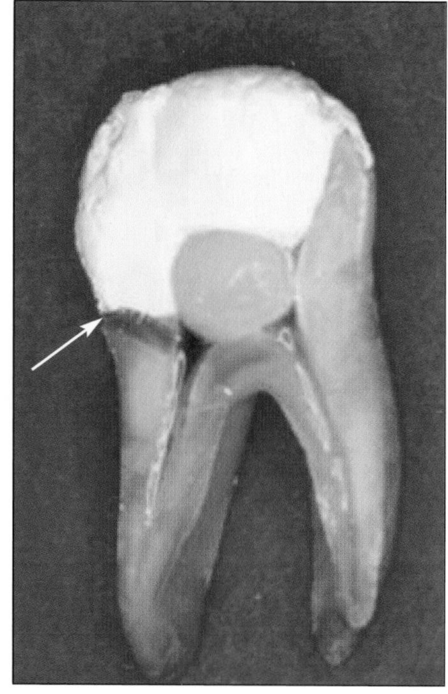

Fig 4-10 Caries left in a tooth during endodontic treatment or after placement of the temporary filling. The primary goal of root canal therapy and microbial control can never be achieved under these circumstances.

2. The access and approximately 2 cm of rubber dam are then disinfected (Fig 4-12). Chlorhexidine and betadine are common medicaments used for this purpose. From this point on, all instruments that enter the canal must be sterile.

Fig 4-11 Removal of caries and leaky restorations and sealing of the rubber dam against saliva contamination.

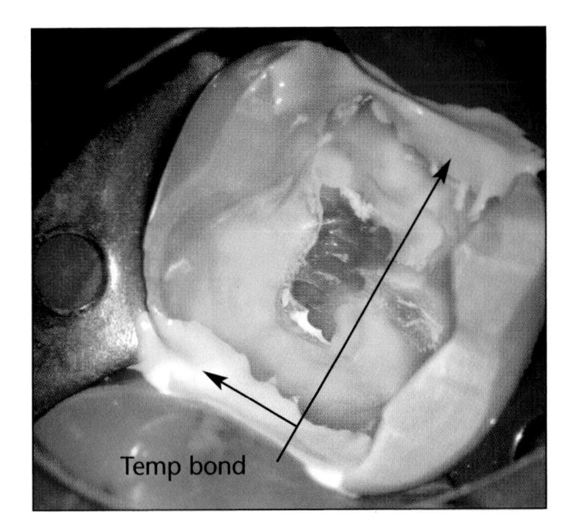

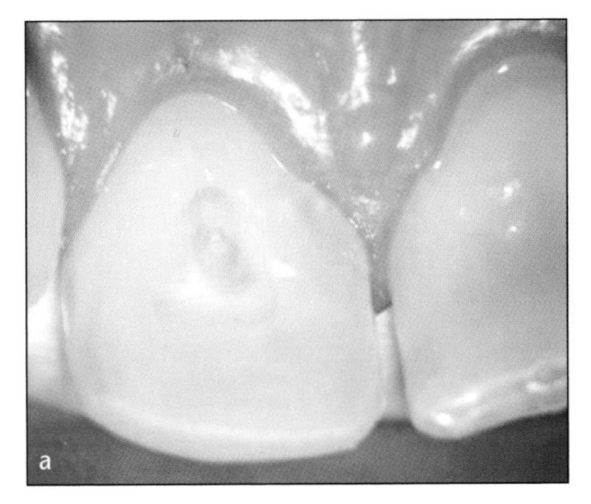

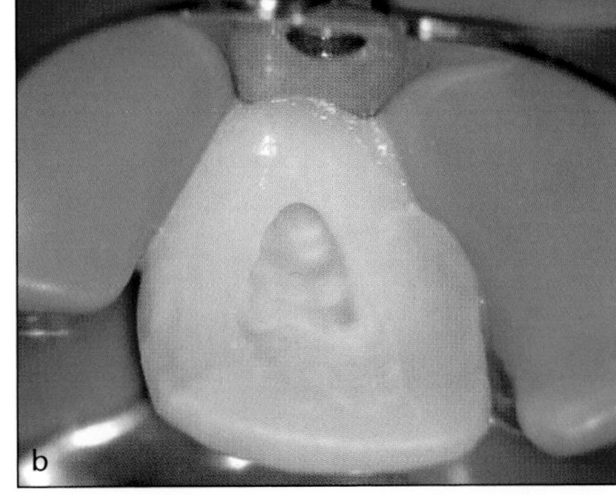

Fig 4-12 Aseptic technique. *(a)* Access without rubber dam. *(b)* Placement of rubber dam. *(c)* Disinfection of the operative field with chlorhexidine or betadine.

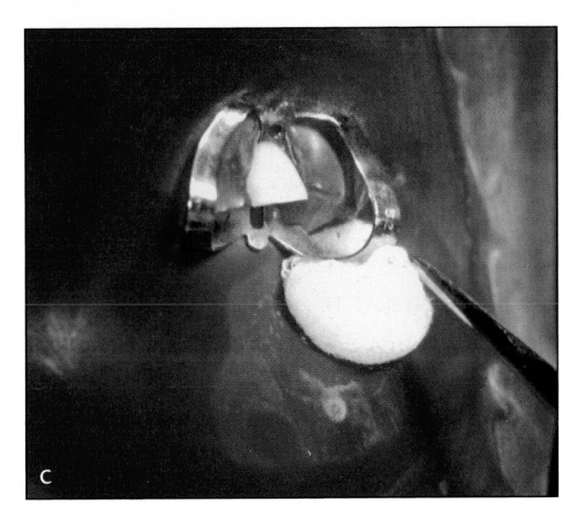

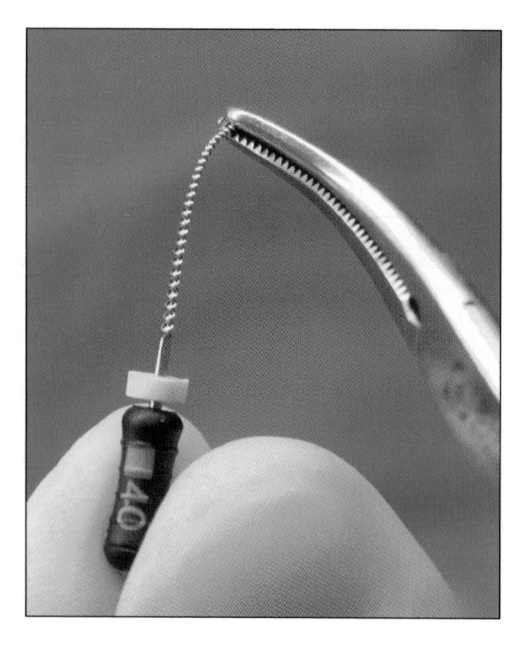

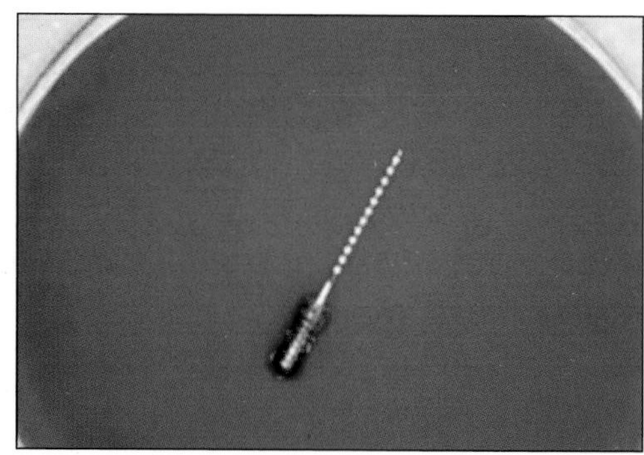

Fig 4-13a Maintaining asepsis by using a sterile hemostat to curve a file *(left)*. When the file is placed in a blood agar plate *(above)*, no growth of microbes occurs.

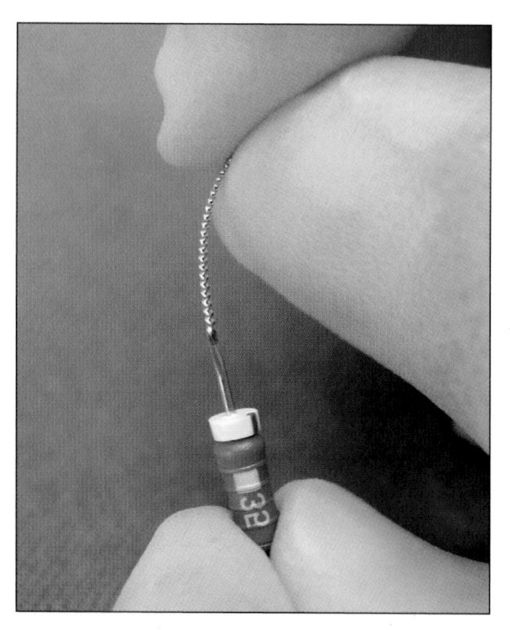

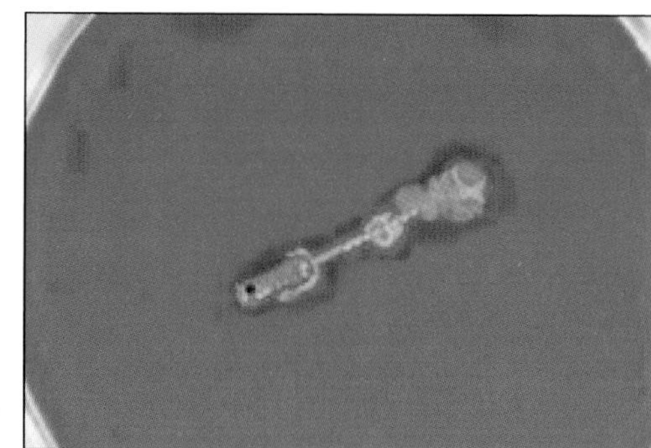

Fig 4-13b When a gloved finger is used to curve the file *(left)*, microbes grow around it in the blood agar plate *(above)*.

3. Divide the work area itself into "dirty" and "clean" areas to maintain sterility. Never touch the files with your hands (Fig 4-13); instead, use sterile cotton pliers or a similar type of instrument.
4. Keep all sterile (clean) instruments to the left and all used (dirty) instruments to the right. A used instrument on the right side must not be reused until it has been disinfected and replaced on the left side (Fig 4-14).

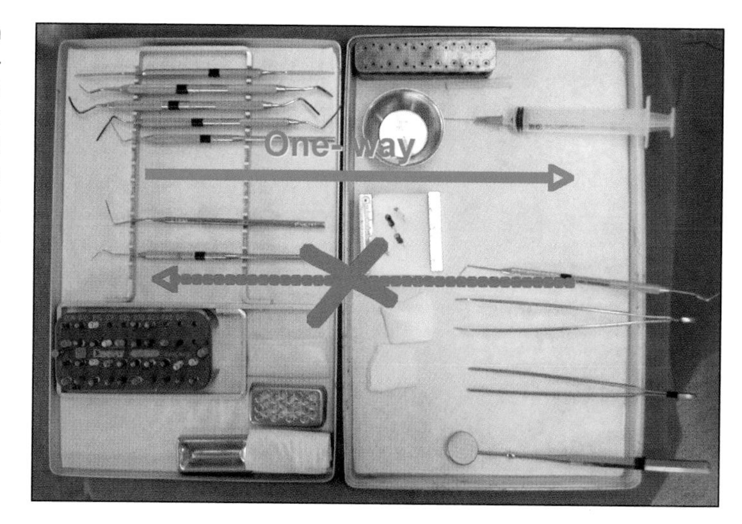

Fig 4-14 To maintain asepsis, all used (dirty) instruments are placed on the right side of the tray. Instruments must be wiped off and sterilized before they can be put back on the left (clean) side of the tray.

Working Length

Even to this day, the length to which the canal should be instrumented remains a controversial topic of discussion. Most clinicians agree that the apical constriction or narrowest point, often referred to as the *minor foramen*, does not correspond to the tip of the root (Fig 4-15). Thus, if the file reaches the radiographic apex, it is very likely to have penetrated the foramen (Fig 4-16). Histologic studies show that the constriction is situated on average about 0.5 mm coronal to the root apex. In addition, outcome studies on root canal treatment conclude that in a tooth with a vital pretreatment diagnosis, the best results are obtained when the canal is instrumented and filled 1 to 2 mm coronal to the radiographic apex.

On the other hand, in a tooth diagnosed with necrotic pulp and apical periodontitis, the best results are expected when the tooth is filled 0.5 to 1 mm coronal to the radiographic apex (Fig 4-17). Nearly all studies show that for both diagnostic categories, a long core fill offers the worst prognosis! It is also important to establish a working length for instrumentation that is at, or short of, the canal minor foramen for root canal filling purposes. By creating a stop at the apex, pressure can be used to place the filling material and to fill the entire canal. In this way, the material can be moved in a lateral direction, thus conforming to the shape of the true canal (Fig 4-18). Filling a canal without a mechanical stop at the apex would be analogous to filling a mesio- or disto-occlusal cavity preparation without having a wedge on the matrix. Material would "leak" into the periodontal ligament, leaving the cavity unfilled and susceptible to re-infection.

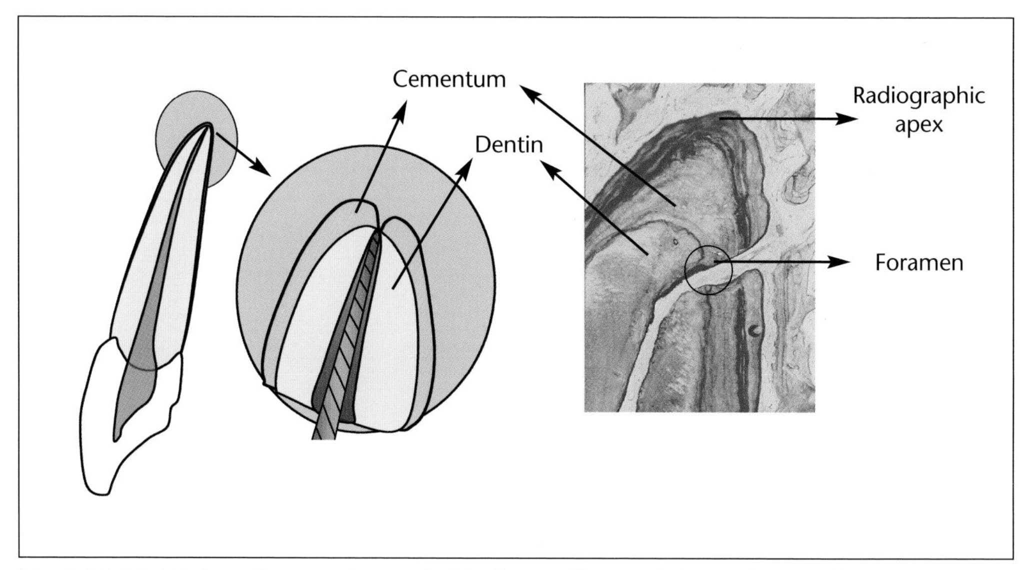

Fig 4-15 Mesial view of an anterior tooth. The "natural" constriction in the apical area is 0.5 to 1.0 mm from the radiographic apex.

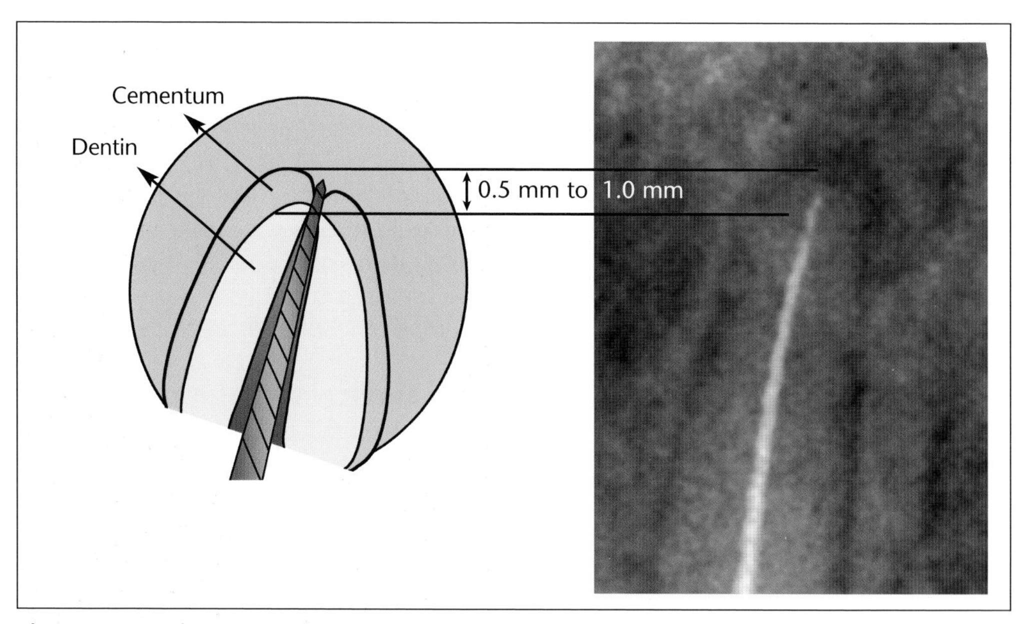

Fig 4-16 Mesial view of an anterior tooth. A radiograph that shows the file at the apex of the root probably means that it has penetrated the apical constriction.

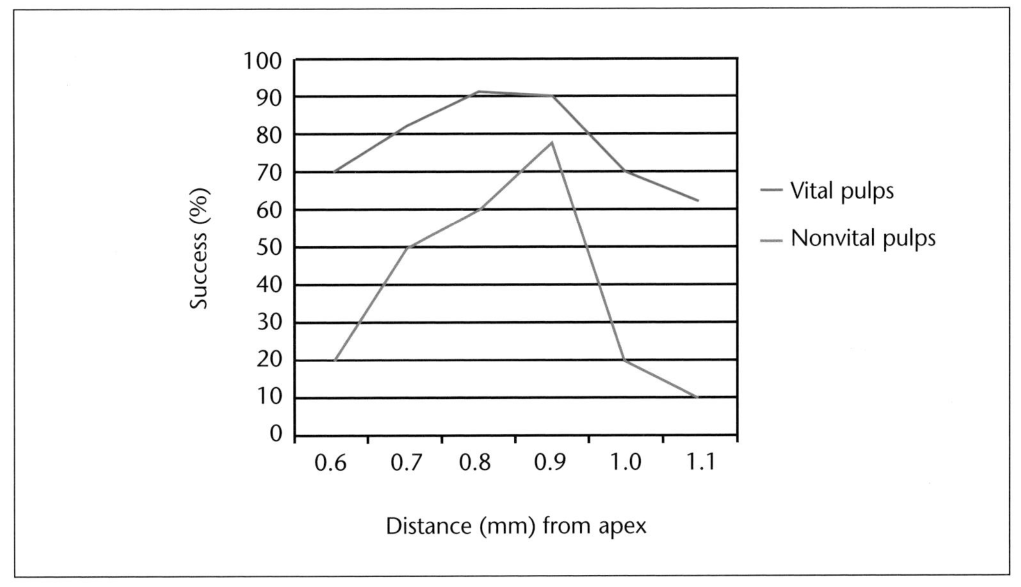

Fig 4-17 Success rates for teeth with (pretreatment) vital and nonvital pulps. For both categories, the highest success rates are achieved when the teeth are filled short of the radiographic apex. Particularly in nonvital teeth, the success rate decreases when the core filling is long.

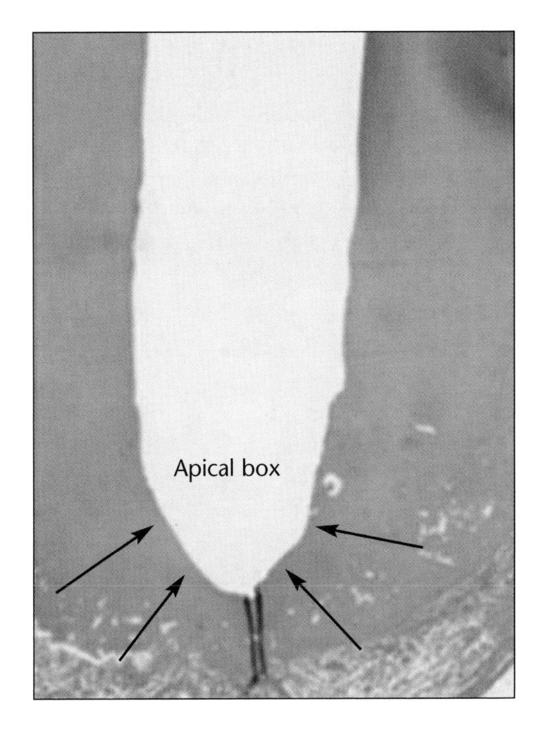

Fig 4-18 The apical box within dentin creates a matrix that enables optimal filling of the space.

At this stage of treatment, it is not necessary to know the precise working length since the length of the canal will change slightly once the coronal two thirds is instrumented. Therefore, a preliminary working length should be established 1 mm from the radiographic measure at this stage of treatment. If the clinician is confident that the preoperative radiograph was taken in a parallel fashion (see Estimated Working Length, above), it is even possible to dispense with the working length radiograph and take an exact length radiograph after the coronal two thirds of the canal have been prepared.

Root Canal Instrumentation

Once all caries and leaky restorations have been removed, straight line access has been attained, and an aseptic environment ensured through the use of a well-sealed rubber dam and surface disinfectant, it is time to instrument the root canals. This is the most important aspect of microbial control and is performed in conjunction with the use of antimicrobial irrigating solutions.

Root canal exploration with a stainless steel no. 10 file is performed prior to taking the working length radiograph. It is important to understand that NiTi instruments merely follow canals; they do not find them. The clinician must first locate a canal and create a patent pathway to the canal foramen, and the NiTi instruments will then easily follow this path. The canals are explored using "stiff" stainless steel files (no. 8, no. 10, no. 15, or no. 20). In the authors' experience, the no. 10 file will most often conform to the estimated working length of the canal. An exploratory curve is placed in the apical 2 to 3 mm of the file (Fig 4-19), allowing the tip to explore a different direction in the canal with a slight twist of the file handle. Using this "watch-winding" motion, the file should "slip and slide" down the canal. If it encounters an obstacle, the file can be retracted slightly, the handle twisted to change the orientation of the tip, and the file can again be advanced to continue exploring the canal (Fig 4-20). Extreme patience and care must be exercised by the clinician when attempting to negotiate an obstacle in the canal. If the file is forced against an obstacle, a ledge is created that will be very difficult to bypass (Fig 4-21).

If the file remains loose in the canal as it nears the estimated working length, larger stainless steel files should be placed to the foramen until a size is reached that cannot easily be placed to the estimated working length. Increasing the size of the "natural" canal now reduces the number of NiTi instruments that will be required later to make the apical third of the canal smaller in diameter than the rest of the canal (see Chapter 3, General Principles). Once the file nears the estimated working length, the crown-down technique can be employed using the rotary instruments.

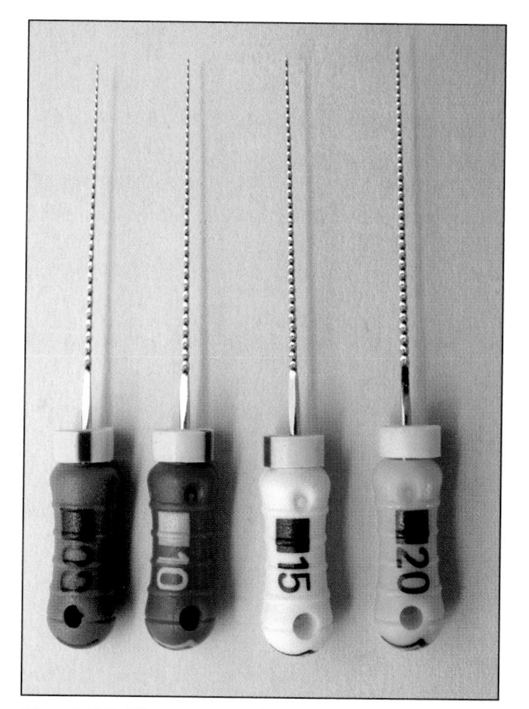

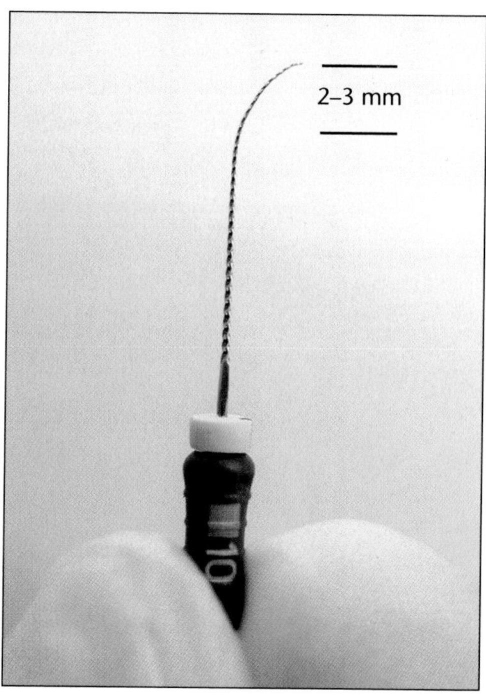

Fig 4-19 Placement of an exploratory curve on a "stiff" stainless steel instrument. The operator slides the instrument down the canal using a "watch winding" motion.

Fig 4-20 Watch-winding motion used to slide the precurved file down the canal.

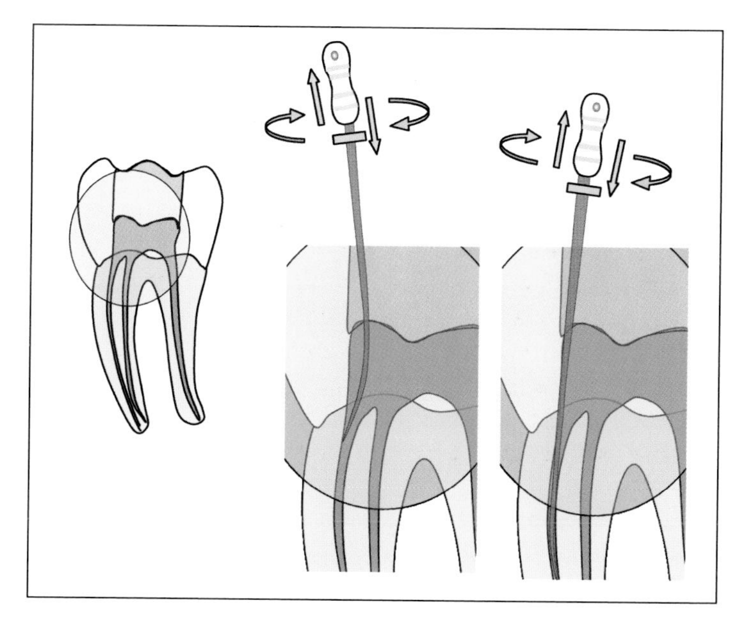

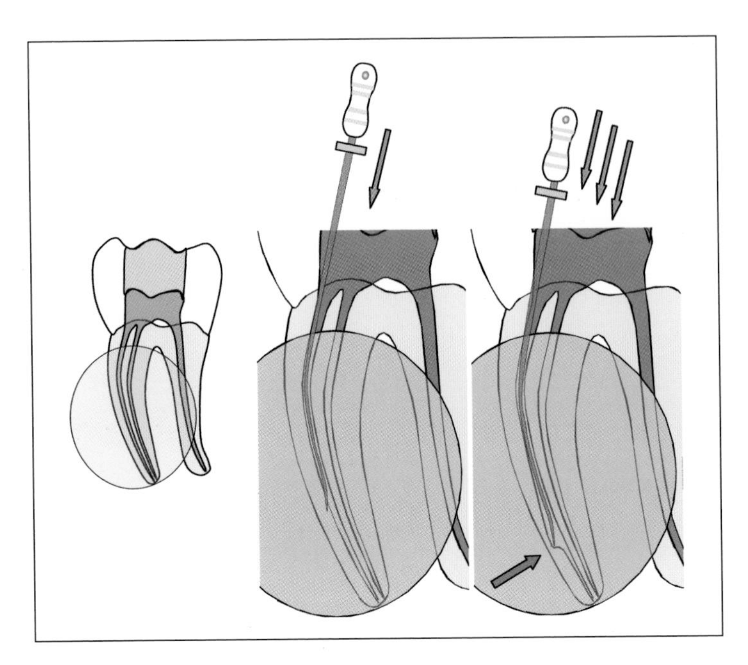

Fig 4-21a Bypassing an obstacle in the canal. If blockage is encountered, it is important not to force the file further into the canal, as this can create a ledge in the canal wall.

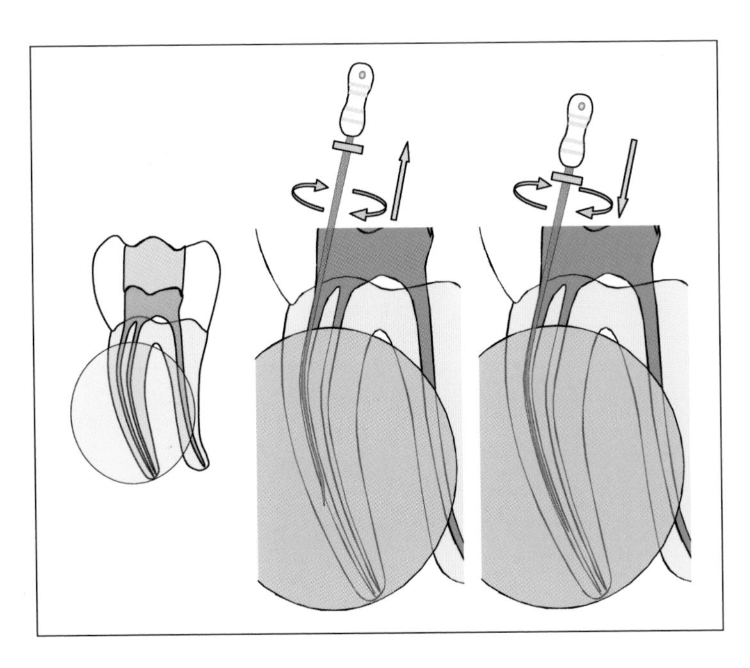

Fig 4-21b Bypassing an obstacle in the canal. The precurved file should be retracted slightly and wound like a watch to change the position of the tip in the canal. An attempt is then made to gently advance the file past the blockage.

Modified step-back technique with stainless steel files

As stated earlier, the use of an apex-to-crown technique with instruments ranging in size from small to large rarely allows the practitioner to reach a size needed to adequately clean the canal. When this technique is employed, the apical part of the canal becomes packed with dentinal debris that block the larger files' pathway to the apical third or, worse still, direct the file away from a curved canal, causing canal straightening, stripping (perforation in the furca), or even apical perforation. To eliminate these problems, the following modified version of the step-back technique was devised:

1. Using stainless steel files in sizes up to no. 25 (or no. 30 if no. 25 is extremely easy), instrument to the working length. Follow with copious irrigation to rinse the canal.
2. Increase the file by one size to no. 30 (or no. 35) and instrument the canal until the file reaches 1 mm short of the working length. Irrigate as before.
3. Repeat the process until the canal coronal to 4 mm from the working length is instrumented with a size no. 40 file.
4. Using an up-and-down filing motion, increase the size of the canal coronal to 4 mm from the working length (ie, to the same point reached in step 3) using a file one size larger than was used to instrument to the 4-mm point.
5. Re-enter the canal with a size no. 30 file all the way to working length. This instrument should reach the working length easily and with minimal friction as a result of the previous instrumentation.
6. Instrument the apical third of the canal until it reaches a biologically acceptable size (Figs 4-22 and 4-23).

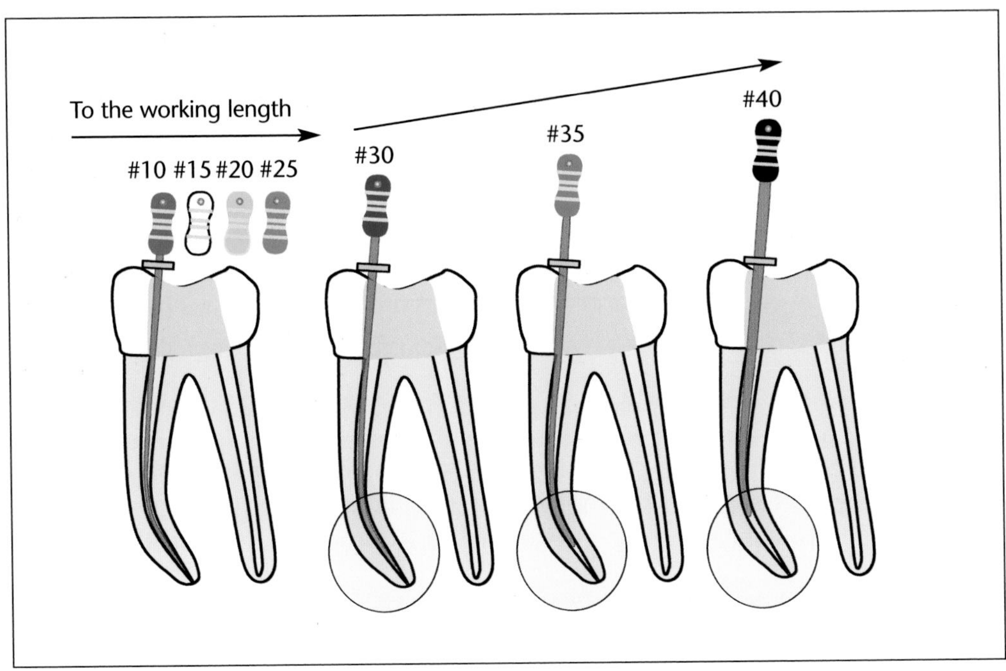

Fig 4-22 Modified step-back technique. Step 1: Space is created in the coronal two thirds of the canal by performing the traditional step-back technique.

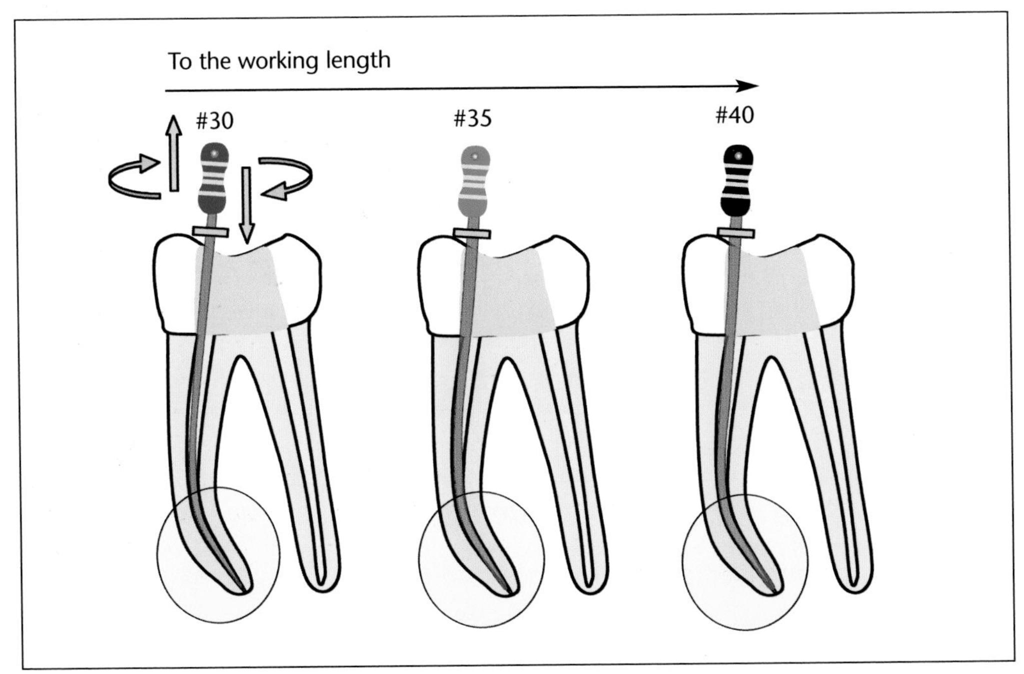

Fig 4-23 Modified step-back technique. Step 2: The apical third of the canal is instrumented to biologic sizes without creating a dentinal plug.

Crown-down technique with NiTi rotary instruments

As noted above, the authors believe that rotary NiTi instruments offer significant advantages over stainless steel files and should be seriously considered by all practitioners. Indeed, instrumentation of the canal using stainless steel instruments exclusively is a topic that should be discussed only in historic terms. NiTi instruments are extremely flexible and can be bent into almost any position. They will spring back to their original (straight) shape as soon as they are removed from the canal. However, it is important to recognize that, despite their flexibility, there is a tendency for NiTi instruments to straighten the canal. The conflict between the flexibility of the instrument (which allows it to maintain the shape of the canal) and its inherent tendency to straighten (which leads to canal straightening) will ultimately depend on the dentin's resistance to being cut versus the instrument's efficiency in cutting. It is extremely important to know the cutting efficiency of each NiTi file since that will determine how it should be used.

"Nonefficient" cutting instruments

Most of the original NiTi rotary instruments may be classified as "nonefficient" (Fig 4-24). Instead of cutting easily into the dentin, these instruments merely plane the walls of the canal. However, this apparent disadvantage is easily compensated for by the handpiece that powers the instrument at speeds of 150 to 2,000 rpm. It is difficult if not impossible to straighten a canal with one of these instruments, making it ideal for clinicians with no prior experience using NiTi files. The only mishap that can occur is fracturing of the file—there is no danger of straightening the canal.

As a practitioner grows more confident in the use of these files, more aggressive instruments may be considered. Recently, a new type of NiTi instrument was introduced, which features acute-angled cutting edges similar to those found on stainless steel files (Figs 4-25 and 4-26). These acute-angled cutting edges make the instruments much more efficient than their predecessors in the cutting of dentin. The advantage, of course, is that they perform their function much more quickly using fewer instruments than the less-efficient NiTi instruments described above. The drawback of these instruments is their capacity to overcome the resistance of the dentin, thereby increasing the operator's risk of straightening the canal. Recognizing the differences between the two types of NiTi files and knowing which type of file is being used is therefore critically important. Regardless of the type being used, the file must never be left rotating in one position in the canal. While the file is advancing or retreating from the apex, there is little risk of straightening the canal. However, when the file is rotating and allowed to remain stationary within the canal, the result will certainly be a straightened canal.

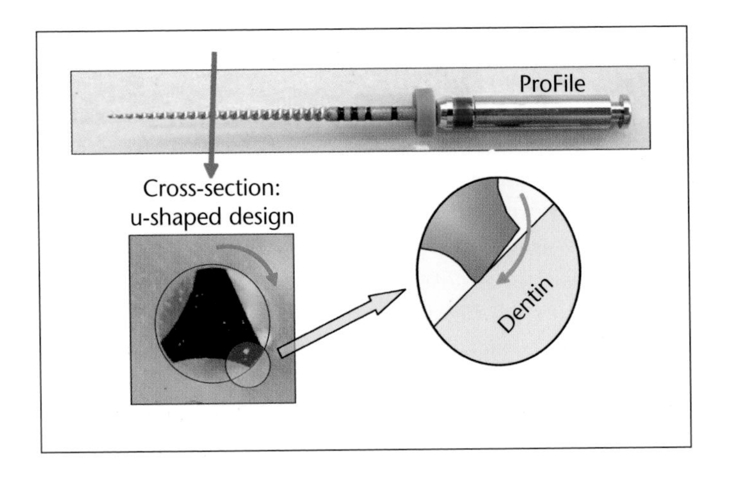

Fig 4-24 ProFile instruments cut inefficiently because of their planing action. This inefficiency guarantees that the canal will not be straightened.

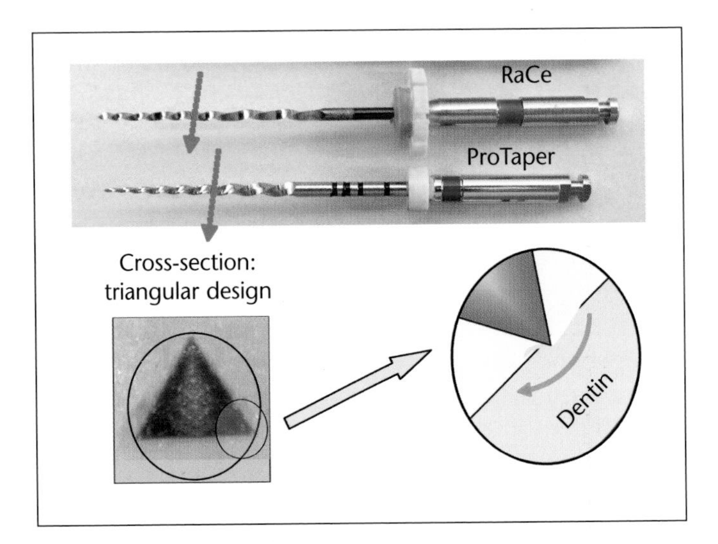

Fig 4-25 ProTaper and RaCe files are efficient cutting instruments because they have acute angles.

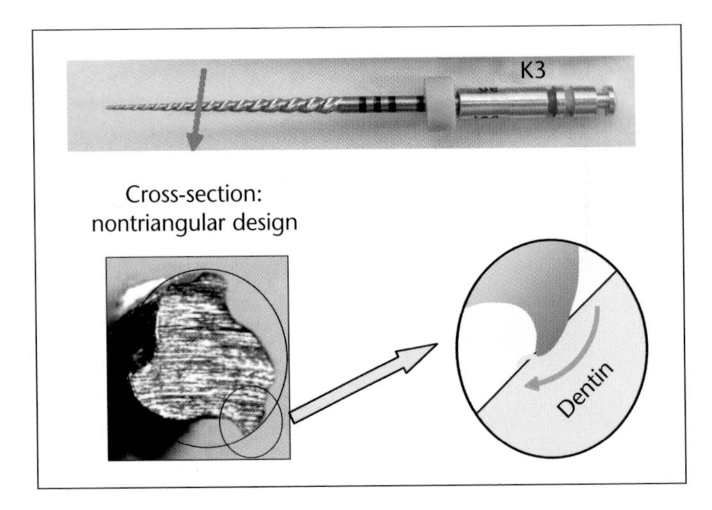

Fig 4-26 K3 also is an efficient cutting file.

There are many NiTi file systems available on the market today, and all of them, in the authors' opinion, are superior to stainless steel files when used correctly. Below is a list of general guidelines for instrumenting a root canal using NiTi files in two steps: a crown-down technique for the coronal two thirds of the canal, followed by a separate step to enlarge the apical third of the canal.

1. Gain straight-line access to the orifices (see Fig 4-19).
2. Explore the canal using stainless steel exploratory files (see Fig 4-20).
3. Instrument the coronal one third of the canal (ie, working length minus 8 mm) with 0.10 followed by 0.08 and then 0.06 tapered instruments of decreasing tip size (but not less than no. 25) (Fig 4-27).
4. Instrument the middle one third of the canal (ie, working length minus 4 mm) with 0.06 and 0.04 instruments with decreasing tip sizes (but not less than no. 25) (Fig 4-28).

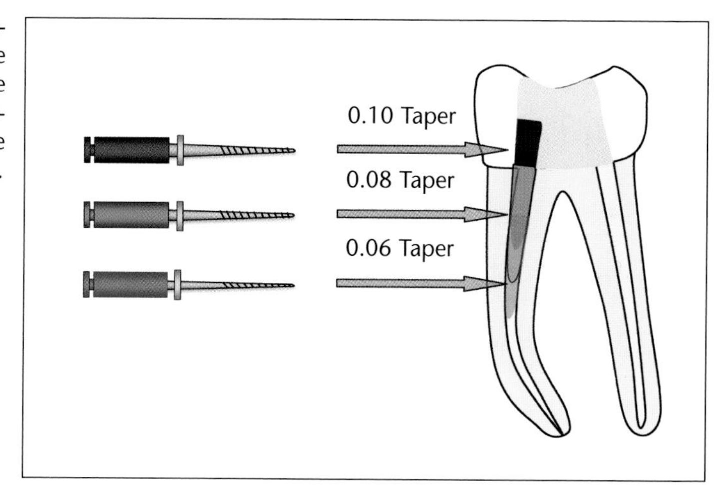

Fig 4-27 Crown-down technique. Preparation of the coronal one third of the canal using files with decreasing taper and, in some systems, decreasing tip sizes.

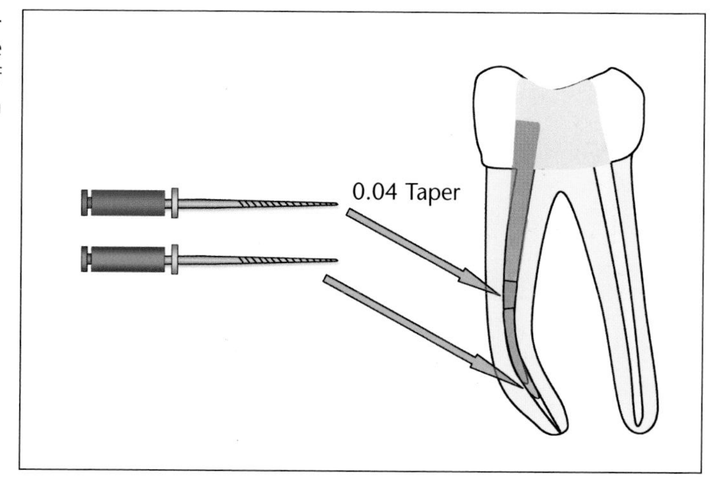

Fig 4-28 Crown-down technique. Continuation of the process with instruments of the same taper but with smaller tip sizes.

Once the coronal two thirds of the canal have been instrumented, determining an accurate working length is imperative since the apical third must be instrumented to the same length with each file. An accurate working length is critical to the success of root canal treatment. For this reason, the authors strongly advise that it be determined only after the coronal two thirds of the canal have been prepared, since this first stage of instrumentation can result in some straightening or shortening of the canal and thereby alter its length.

A number of different methods can be used to determine the correct working length. Using all of them will significantly increase the chances that the instrument length chosen is the correct one.

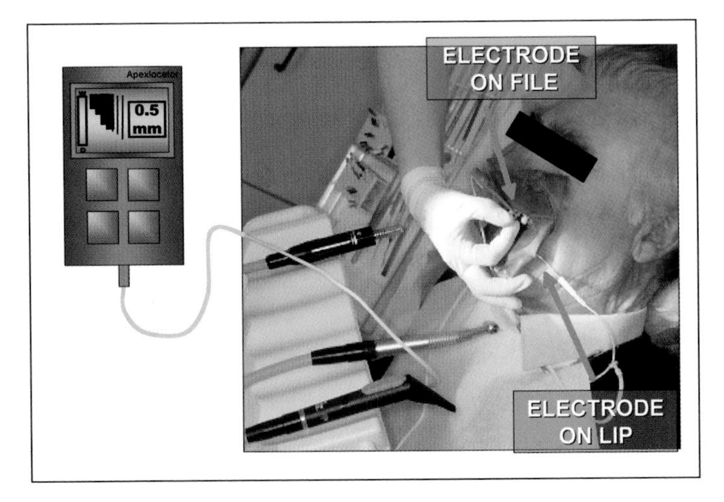

Fig 4-29 The apex locator is one of the most accurate methods available for locating the canal constriction. The electrode is attached to the lip and then the circuit is completed when the second electrode is attached to the file.

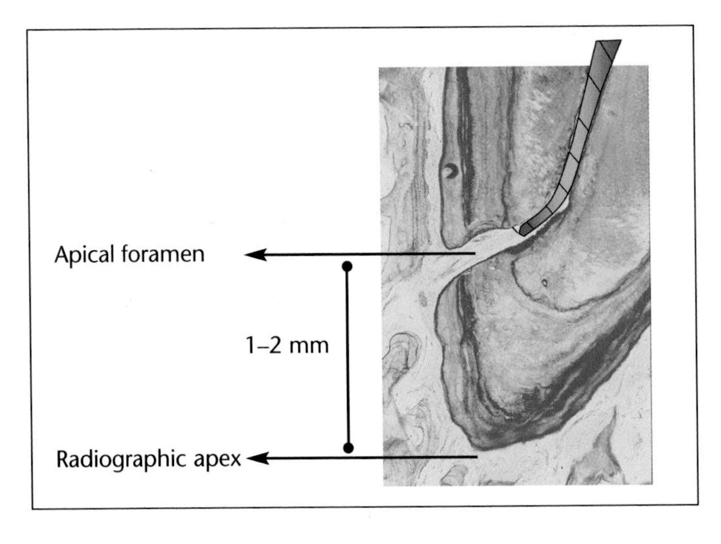

Fig 4-30 The canal constriction is located at a distance that usually falls short of the radiographic apex.

- Digital feel. Since the coronal two thirds of the canal has already been prepared, it is possible to gauge the size and position of the minor foramen using a small file. A no. 10 file can be placed at the estimated working length; if the file slips past the estimated working length, the file size is too small. Thus, it should be increased until the file hits a "dead stop" close to the estimated working length. Most of the time this dead stop length is the accurate working length.
- Electronic apex locator (Figs 4-29 to 4-31). There are numerous electronic apex locators on the market, most of them accurate and able to work in the presence of some moisture. In the authors' view, this instrument is a valuable tool that should be used in most cases. When following the file's movement toward and away from the minor foramen, this instrument is the most accurate indicator of canal length available.

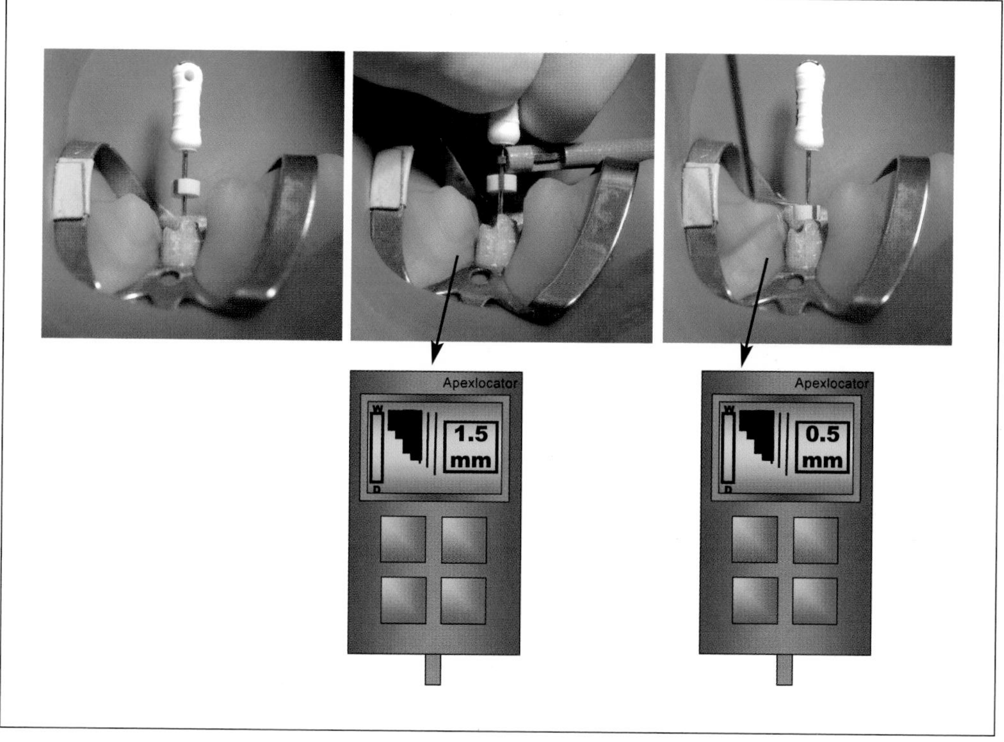

Fig 4-31 The apex locator will start to register a length about 1.5 mm from the apical constriction. In most cases, the length is deemed acceptable when the machine registers 0.5 mm from the apical constriction. If movement of the file between two lengths (1.5 mm and 0.5 mm) registers a corresponding change in the apex locator indicator, the machine is assumed to be accurate.

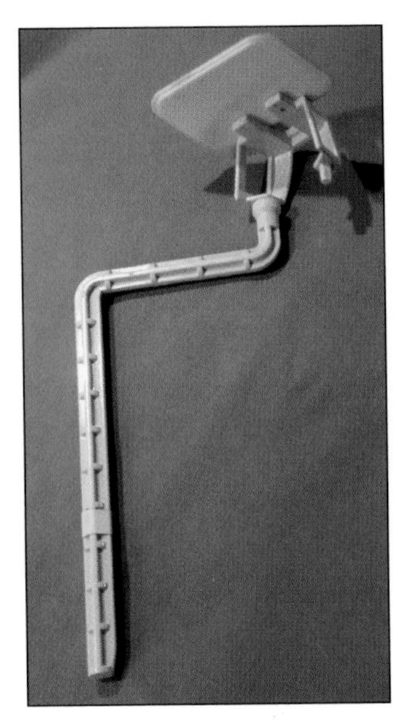

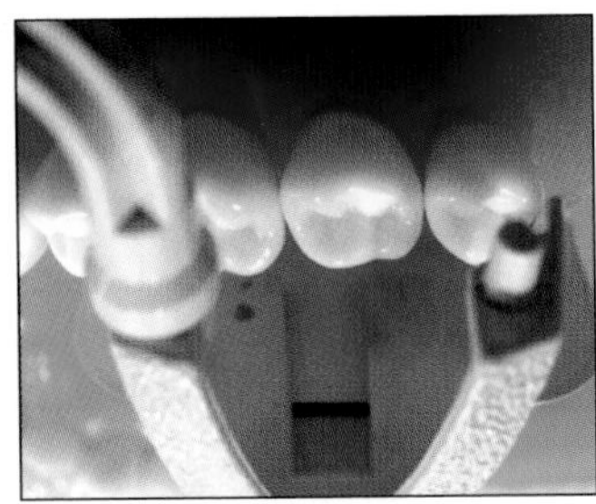

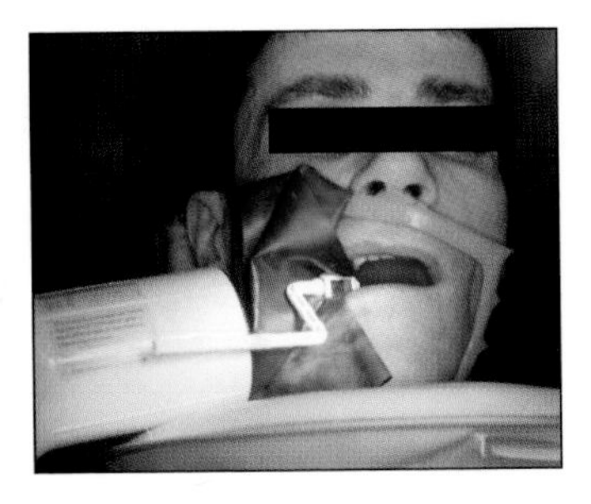

Fig 4-32 A radiographic paralleling device allows a parallel radiograph to be taken with the endodontic files in place.

- Radiograph. A radiograph is the most common means of determining working length. Radiographic paralleling devices (see Estimated Working Length, above) can be used in conjunction with files placed in the tooth (Fig 4-32). However, it is important to recognize that the working length as measured on a radiograph is only an estimate, and therefore digital feel and an apex locator should also be used to confirm the accuracy of the working length.

Once an accurate working length has been determined, rotary NiTi files with ISO sizes 15 to 80 and a taper of 0.02 or 0.04 are used to the appropriate size to maximize the chances of effectively cleaning the canal (Fig 4-33).

- Sizes 15 and over are manually advanced into the canal in progressive succession to identify the instrument that does not reach the accurate working length, usually no. 20 or no. 25.
- The apical third of the canal is then prepared with successively larger sizes until the appropriate size has been reached.

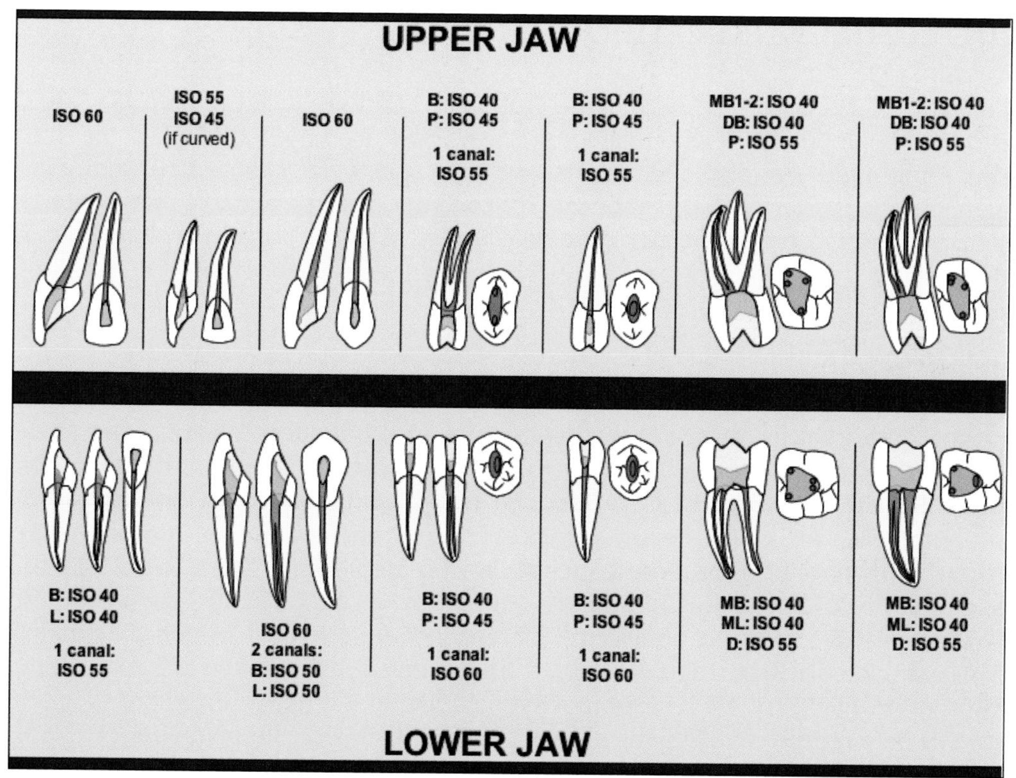

Fig 4-33a Minimum sizes of last apical instrument in root canal instrumentation.

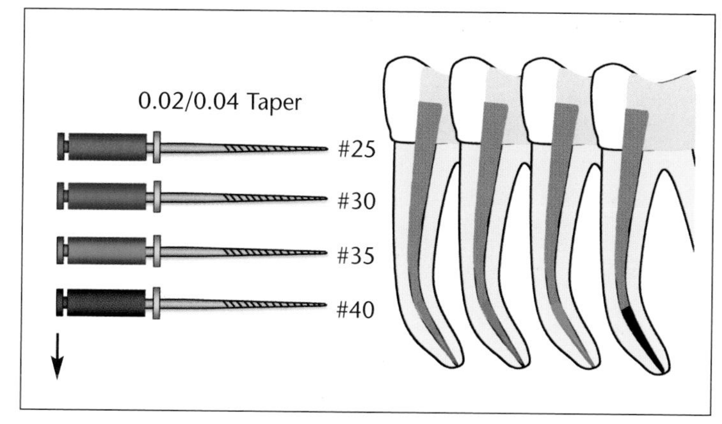

Fig 4-33b Crown-down technique. After the coronal two thirds of the canal has been prepared, the apical one third is prepared to biologic sizes with successively larger files.

Intracanal Medication

Before the canal is filled, intracanal medication is used to reduce the microbial count and thereby optimize the potential for success. While instrumentation plays the most critical role in the microbial control phase of root canal therapy, intracanal medication is an important adjunct that is necessary for consistent and predictable disinfection of the canals. Intracanal medications can be classified as either irrigating solutions or as medications that remain inside the canal between visits.

Irrigants

Sodium hypochlorite is the most popular intracanal irrigating solution currently in use. It is both antimicrobial and able to break down tissue, which is useful in vital cases. Household bleach is 5.25% sodium hypochlorite, which is considered "full strength" for root canal therapy purposes. Many variations in the use of sodium hypochlorite have been proposed, such as varying the strength (0.5% to 5.25%), the temperature, and the length of time it is left inside the canal. However, none of these factors appears to make a significant difference. Sodium hypochlorite is self-limiting in its antimicrobial action and therefore must be replenished as often as is reasonable. Thus, using a 0.5% solution of sodium hypochlorite that is replenished after every file use will be more effective than heating 5.25% sodium hypochlorite to 60°C (107.6°F) and leaving it in the canal for 30 minutes. Sodium hypochlorite can be used very safely if it "passively" washes the canal. It should never be forced through the apex or into the periapical tissues under pressure. When used in this manner, it is highly toxic and will necrotize the periapical tissues. It is therefore critical that the needle is never wedged into the canal but left loose before the medicament is expressed.

Ethylenediaminetetraacetic acid (17% EDTA) is an effective chelating agent often used in conjunction with sodium hypochlorite to remove the smear layer left behind by instrumentation (Fig 4-34). EDTA itself is not antimicrobial; in removing the smear layer, however, it does effectively eliminate the microorganisms residing there. More-

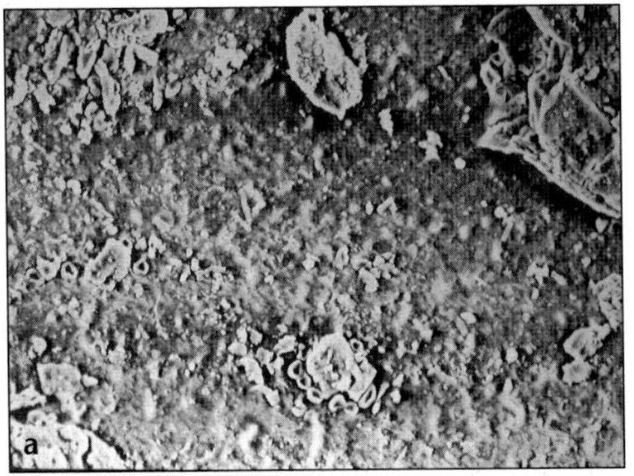

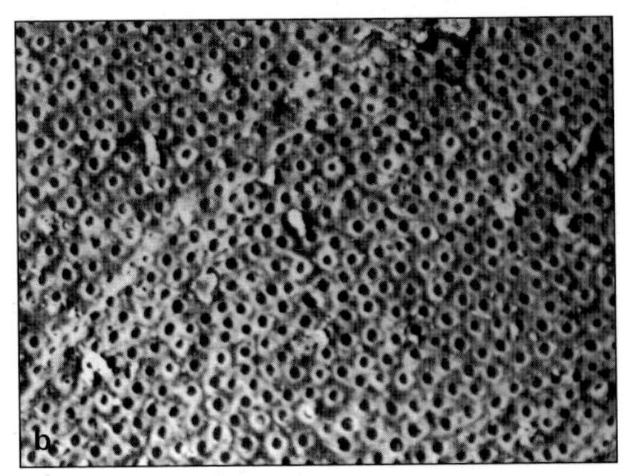

Fig 4-34 Irrigation with sodium hypochlorite alone *(a)* will not remove the smear layer on the canal wall. The addition of 17% EDTA *(b)* is more effective in removing the smear layer, leaving open dentinal tubules.

over, removal of the smear layer increases the effectiveness of other antimicrobial medicaments within the dentinal tubules. EDTA is applied in the same general manner as sodium hypochlorite, and the two are often used as alternating rinses.

Chlorhexidine (2% chlorhexidine) in water is another effective medicament against root canal microbes. An advantage of this medicament is that it adheres (substantively) to the canal walls, which extends its action for a few days to several weeks. However, it lacks the tissue-dissolving property of sodium hypochlorite. Chlorhexidine also can be use in conjunction with EDTA.

Interappointment medication

Calcium hydroxide ($Ca[OH]_2$) is a medicament used between visits to decrease the microbial count to a level that will guarantee a high rate of success following canal- and crown-filling procedures. $Ca(0H)_2$ should be used routinely in nonvital infected cases and in vital cases when instrumentation and filling cannot be completed within a single visit. $Ca(OH)_2$ powder is mixed with sterile saline or 2% chlorhexidine in water to achieve a creamy toothpaste-like consistency. Using a lentulo-spiral instrument, it is then spun into the prepared canal until it reaches within 2 mm of the working length (Figs 4-35 and 4-36). Commercially prepared soft $Ca(0H)_2$ products are also useful for root canal disinfection.

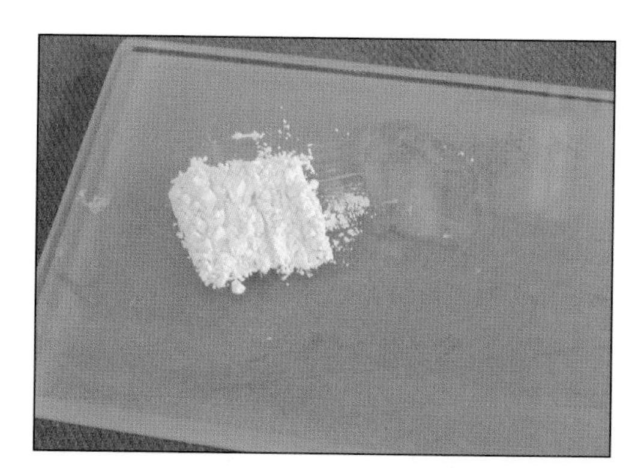
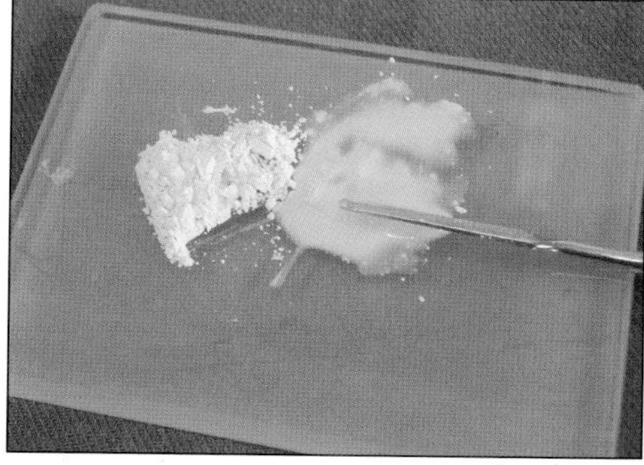

Fig 4-35 Calcium hydroxide powder mixed with saline.

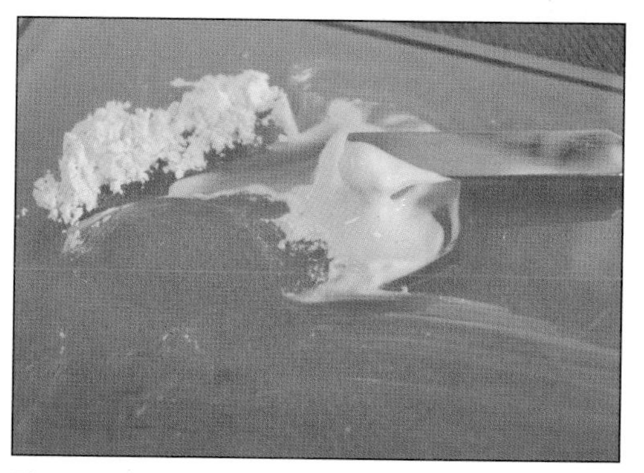
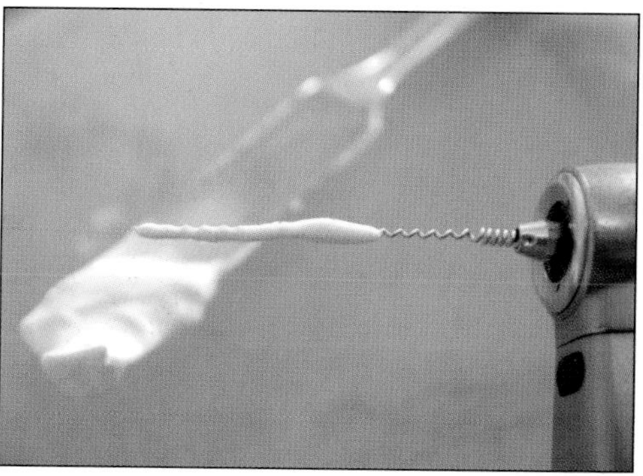

Fig 4-36 The creamy calcium hydroxide is spun into the canal with a lentulo-spiral instrument.

Root Canal Filling

After the microbial control phase is complete, the canal must be filled and sealed. When it is considered appropriate to fill the root canal system, it is also appropriate to place a permanent restoration over it. This coronal restoration is thought to be just as important as the root canal system filling in maintaining an environment that, over time, will result in a healthy periodontium. In creating a hermetic seal in the root canal, the root filling performs three primary functions.

- It entombs remaining microbes in the root canal so that they cannot communicate with the surrounding periodontal ligament to prolong or introduce disease
- It seals out tissue fluids that supply nutrients to the microbes residing in the root canal
- It seals the root canal against microbes communicated via coronal leakage of the saliva.

In addition, the material used to fill the root canals also should have several important properties, including ease of handling, radiopacity, selective toxicity (toxic to microbes in the root canal but not to the periapical tissues when properly applied), and the capacity to be retreated.

Gutta-percha in conjunction with a sealant has been used for many years as the standard root canal filling material. While gutta-percha fulfils most of the secondary functions of a suitable root filling material, it creates a poor seal. Studies have demonstrated conclusively that gutta-percha does not effectively entomb all of the microbes remaining in the canal. In addition, other studies show that gutta-percha and sealant fail miserably in inhibiting coronal leakage. In fact, population studies suggest that the coronal or top filling is critical for periapical health, illustrating the weakness of the gutta-percha filling to seal out oral microbes if the top filling is defective. **Gutta-percha plus sealant represent the weak link in endodontic therapy.**

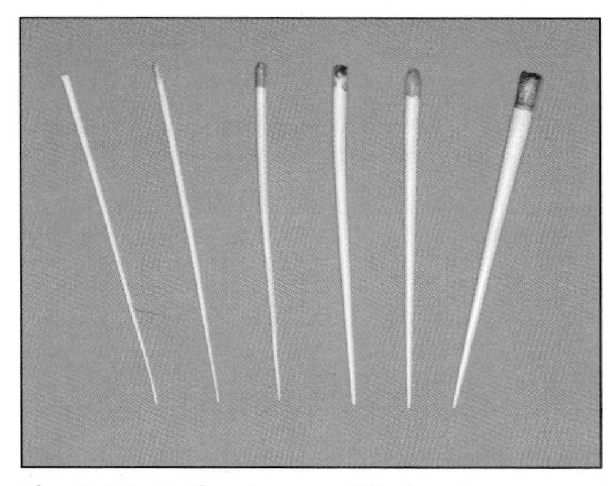

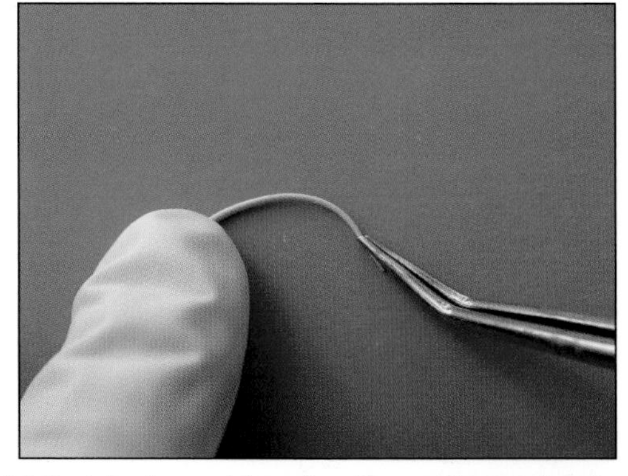

Fig 4-37 Resilon is a modified resin core material that looks and handles like gutta-percha. In addition, fillers have been added to the resin core and sealant that make them retreatable with heat and/or a solvent (Fig 4-38).

An adhesive root filling system designed to replace gutta-percha was recently developed. The Resilon System consists of a modified resin core material (Fig 4-37) that possesses many of the same properties as gutta-percha (Fig 4-38), including the ability to be thermoplasticized.

Resilon points are dimensionally stable since they consist of fully polymerized and cross-linked resin. When thermoplasticized, the resin maintains its cross-linkages but shrinks upon cooling by 0.5% (compared to gutta-percha's 3% to 7% shrinkage). The root filling is completed with the use of a self-etching primer (Fig 4-39) to remove the smear layer from the canal walls and to wet the root canal surface. The self-etching primer has a low surface tension and is hydrophilic in nature. A dual-curable sealant (see Fig 4-39) is then placed into the canal; this sealant bonds to the canal wall and the resin core material, creating a monoblock that for the first time truly seals the canal (Fig 4-40).

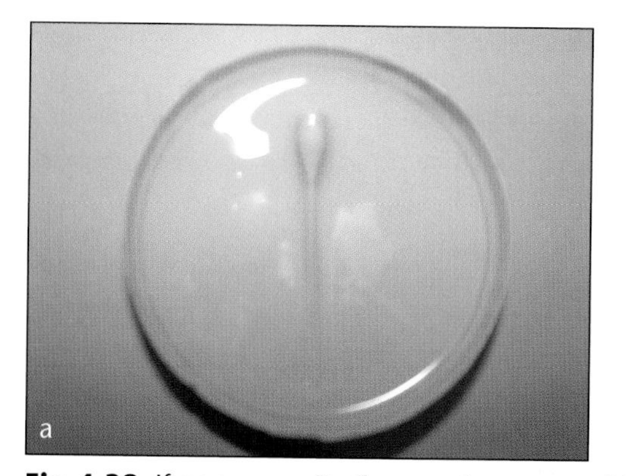

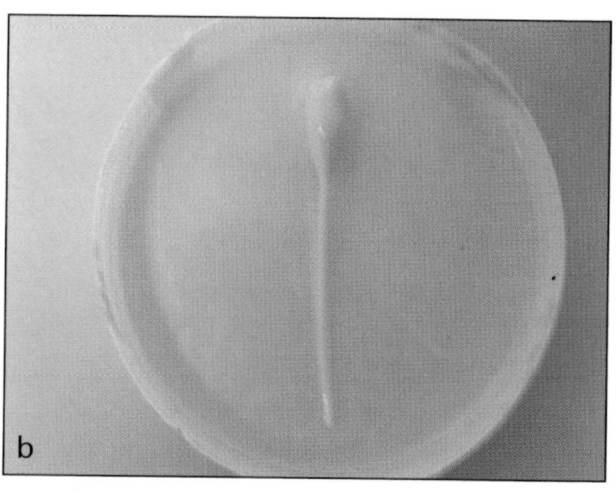

Fig 4-38 If necessary, Resilon can be removed from the root canal with heat and/or solvents. *(a)* Resilon. *(b)* Resilon with chloroform.

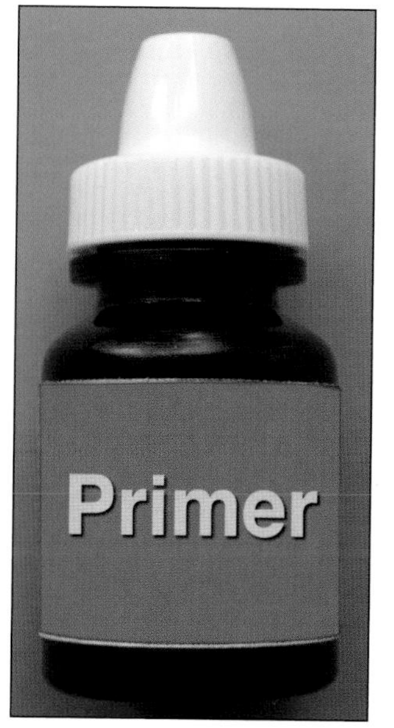

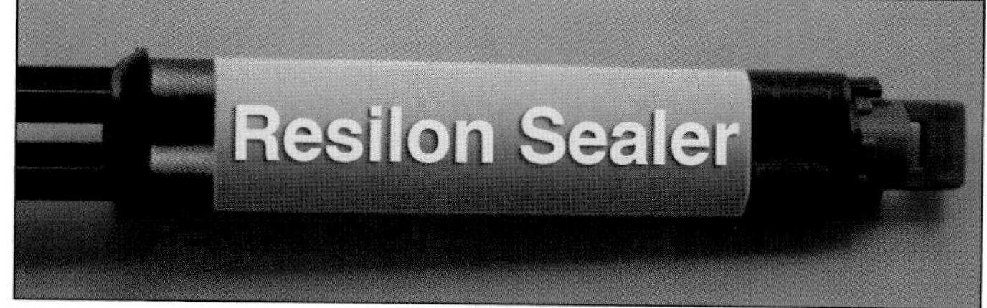

Fig 4-39 The self-etching primer will remove the smear layer and wet the root canal surface, thus lowering the surface tension. The dual-cure resin sealant will bind the resin core material to the canal walls, creating a monoblock.

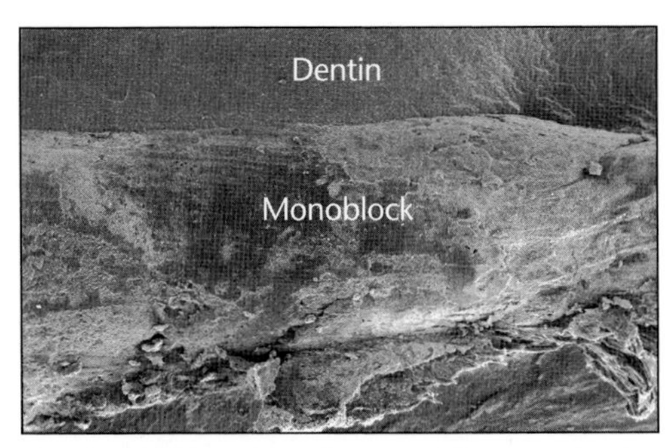

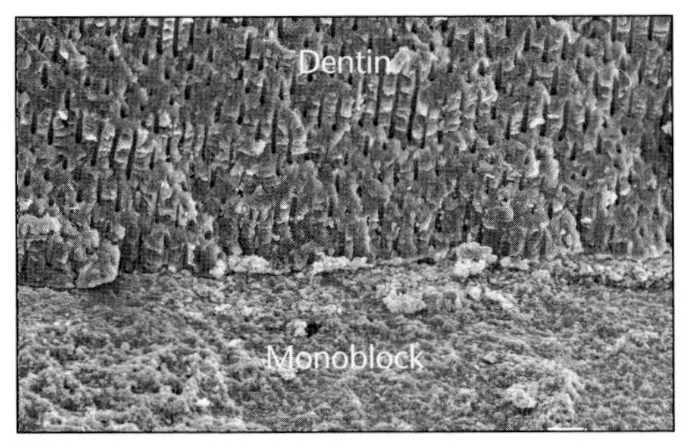

Fig 4-40 Scanning electron micrograph view of the dual-cure resin sealant to the resin core material and to the dentin surface, creating a tight seal against microbial leakage.

Clinical protocol for root canal filling

1. Once the canal has been prepared, EDTA should be used for the final irrigation to remove the smear layer and negate the effect of the NaOCl on the resin bond. Chlorhexidine, which does not affect bond strength, may be added prior to placing the primer (Fig 4-41).
2. Paper points are used to dry the canal, and then an appropriate Resilon master point is placed into the canal. A radiograph is taken to assess whether the Resilon point adapted to the proper apical level. One drop of primer for each canal is dispensed onto a mixing pad. A paper point is soaked in the primer and then placed to length in the canal. Excess primer is dried using additional paper points (Fig 4-42).
3. Next, the sealant is dispensed onto a mixing pad, and, if desired, thinning resin can be added to it to adjust the sealant's viscosity. The Resilon point is coated with sealant, which is then painted on the root canal walls (Fig 4-43).
4. A spreader is used under gentle pressure to create a space between the Resilon point and the canal wall, and an accessory point (FM or MF) covered with sealant is placed into this space. This procedure is repeated until the canal has been filled. A warm stopper is used to sear off the master and accessory points, followed by gentle vertical condensation using a cold stopper (Fig 4-44). Lateral condensation with Resilon generally creates a much lower force than gutta-percha. Although only the lateral condensation technique is described here, all of the thermoplasticized techniques are possible with Resilon. In general, the temperature for adequate flow of Resilon is approximately 30°C lower than for gutta-percha, but each machine should be fine-tuned before use.
5. When root filling is complete, the coronal surface of the root filling may be light-cured for 40 seconds over the pulp chamber, resulting in an immediate coronal seal. Although the resin "monoblock" creates a coronal seal, the final restoration should be placed as soon as possible (Fig 4-45).

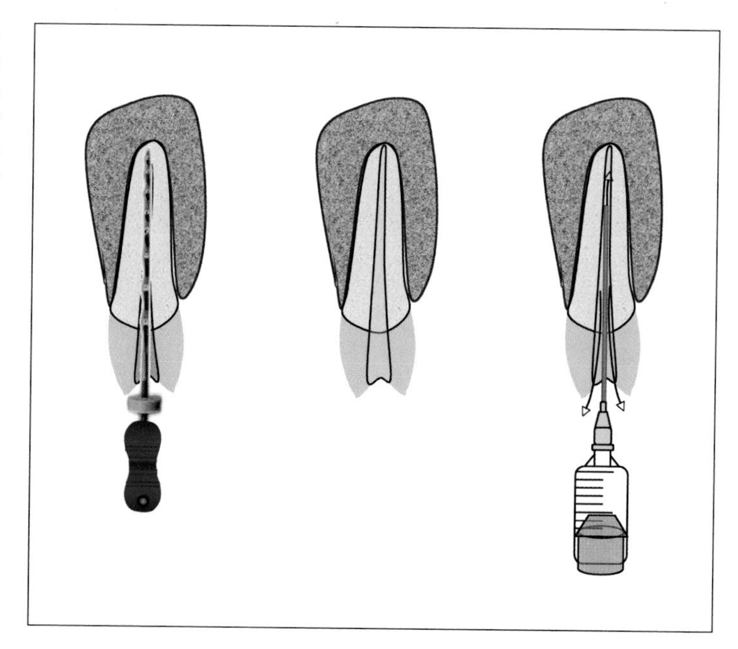

Fig 4-41 The instrumentation is completed with irrigation that may include sodium hypochlorite. For the final irrigation, EDTA and/or 2% chlorhexidine should be used.

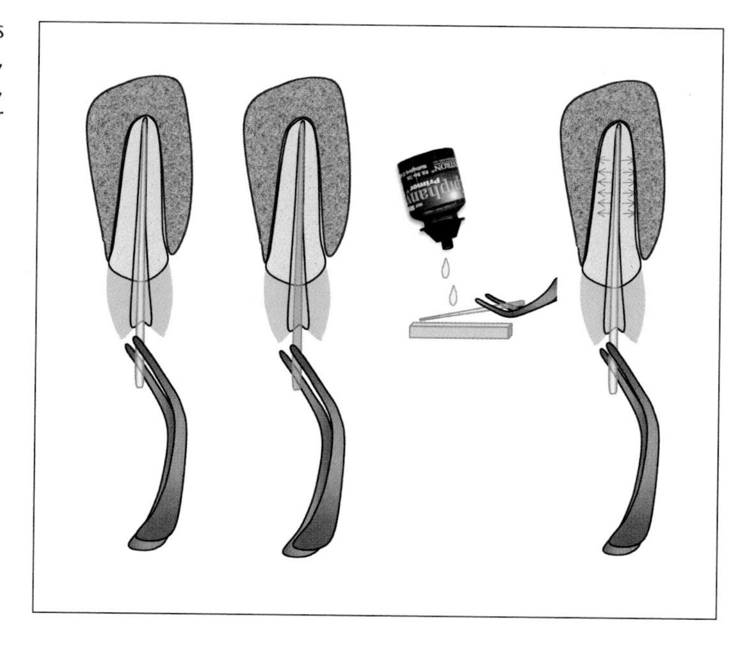

Fig 4-42 The canal is dried with a paper point, the Resilon cone fitted, and a primer-soaked paper point placed to length.

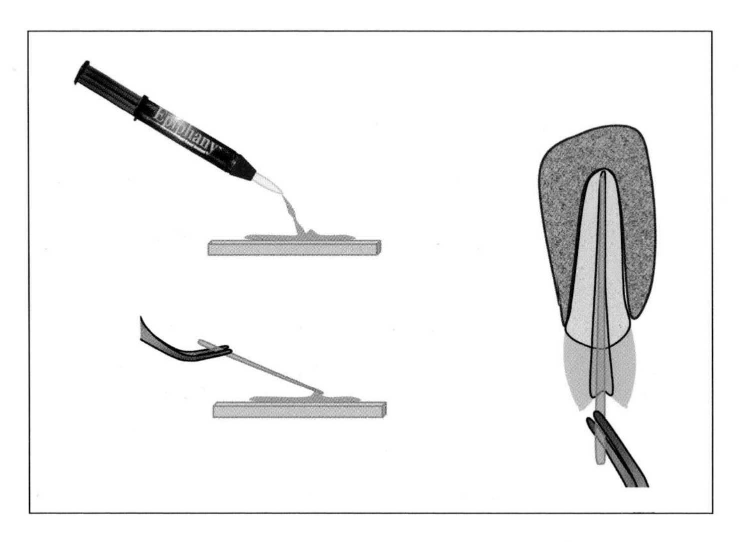

Fig 4-43 The dual-cure sealant is dispensed onto a mixing pad, which is then used to coat the fitted Resilon point. The root canal walls are "painted" with the sealant.

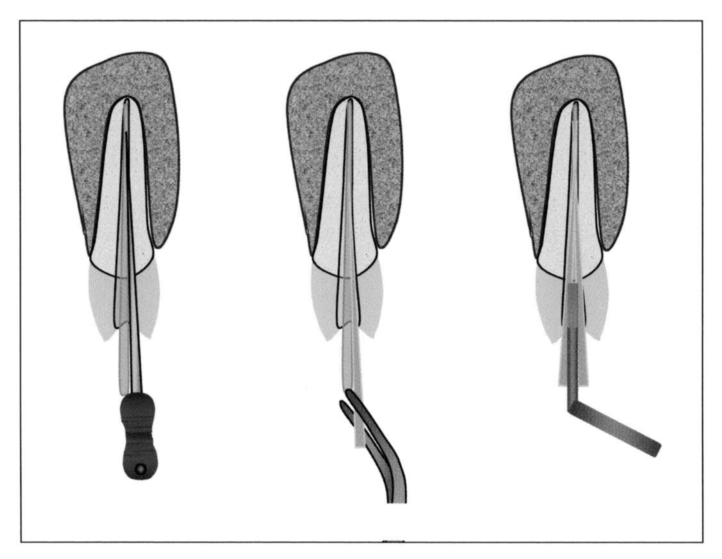

Fig 4-44 Lateral condensation with Resilon. A spreader is used with gentle pressure to explore for space between the master Resilon point and the canal wall. An accessory point covered with sealant is placed into the canal to take up this space. The process is repeated until no more core material can easily be placed into the canal. The excess material is seared off with a hot instrument, and a cold plugger is used to vertically condense the filling material.

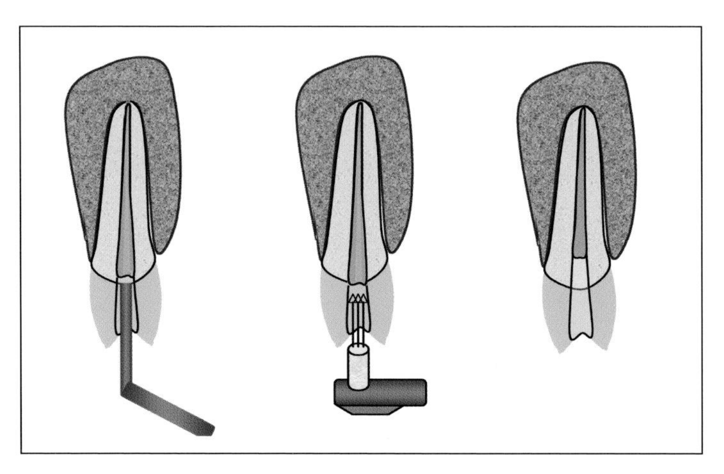

Fig 4-45 After the excess material is removed to the level of the canal orifice, the sealant may be light-cured for 40 seconds to create an immediate coronal seal. The final coronal restoration should be made as soon as possible.

Suggested Reading

1. Hasselgren G, Kerekes K, Nellestram P. pH changes in calcium hydroxide-covered dentin. J Endod 1987; 8:502–505.
2. Kerekes K, Tronstad L. Long-term results of endodontic treatment performed with a standardized technique. J Endod 1979;5:83–90.
3. Leonardo MR, Silva LAB, Almeida WA, Utrilla LS. Tissue response to an epoxy resin-based root canal sealer. Endod Dent Traumatol 1999;15:28–32.
4. Shipper G, Ørstavik D, Teixeira FB, Trope M. An evaluation of microbial leakage in roots filled with a thermoplastic synthetic polymer-based root canal filling material (Resilon). J Endod 2004;30:342–347.
5. Sundqvist G, Figdor D. Endodontic treatment of apical periodontitis. In: Ørstavik D, Pitt Ford TR (eds). Essential Endodontology: Prevention and Treatment of Apical Periodontitis. Oxford: Blackwell-Munksgaard, 1998:242–277.
6. Tronstad L. Clinical Endodontics. 2nd ed. Stuttgart: Thieme, 2003:167–177.
7. Vertucci F. Root canal anatomy of human permanent teeth. Oral Surg Oral Med Oral Pathol 1984;58: 589–597.

5 Treatment Outcome and Prognosis of Endodontic Therapy

It goes without saying that a root canal procedure should be attempted only if the clinician is confident of achieving the highest probability of success for that particular tooth. In order to ensure the best possible outcome, it is essential that only cases that can be performed optimally should be started, whereas more complex cases should be referred to a specialist. In addition, the clinician should know the reported success rate of root canal therapy of teeth with various pulpal diagnoses so that an informed choice of treatment plan can be made.

It is difficult to formulate hard and fast rules regarding which cases to attempt and which to refer because every clinician has a different level of competency. In the authors' opinion, new technologies allow dentists to attempt more and more cases that are reasonable. In theory, as long as the canal can be followed with a small stainless steel exploratory file, it should be possible to enlarge and clean the canal with a rotary file system.

The American Association of Endodontists has devised the following Case Difficulty Assessment Forms and Guidelines (printed with permission of the AAE) to help the dentist decide which cases to treat and which to refer to a specialist.

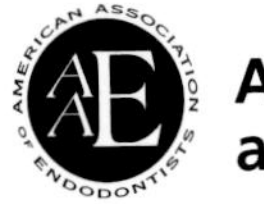

AAE Endodontic Case Difficulty Assessment Form and Guidelines

PATIENT INFORMATION

Name____________________

Address____________________

City/State/Zip____________________

Phone____________________

DISPOSITION

Treat in Office: Yes ☐ No ☐

Refer Patient to:

____

Date:____________________

Guidelines for Using the AAE Endodontic Case Difficulty Assessment Form

The AAE designed the Endodontic Case Difficulty Assessment Form for use in endodontic curricula. The Assessment Form makes case selection more efficient, more consistent and easier to document. Dentists may also choose to use the Assessment Form to help with referral decision making and record keeping.

Conditions listed in this form should be considered potential risk factors that may complicate treatment and adversely affect the outcome. Levels of difficulty are sets of conditions that may not be controllable by the dentist. Risk factors can influence the ability to provide care at a consistently predictable level and impact the appropriate provision of care and quality assurance.

The Assessment Form enables a practitioner to assign a level of difficulty to a particular case.

LEVELS OF DIFFICULTY

MINIMAL DIFFICULTY — Preoperative condition indicates routine complexity (uncomplicated). These types of cases would exhibit only those factors listed in the MINIMAL DIFFICULTY category. Achieving a predictable treatment outcome should be attainable by a competent practitioner with limited experience.

MODERATE DIFFICULTY — Preoperative condition is complicated, exhibiting one or more patient or treatment factors listed in the MODERATE DIFFICULTY category. Achieving a predictable treatment outcome will be challenging for a competent, experienced practitioner.

HIGH DIFFICULTY — Preoperative condition is exceptionally complicated, exhibiting several factors listed in the MODERATE DIFFICULTY category or at least one in the HIGH DIFFICULTY category. Achieving a predictable treatment outcome will be challenging for even the most experienced practitioner with an extensive history of favorable outcomes.

Review your assessment of each case to determine the level of difficulty. If the level of difficulty exceeds your experience and comfort, you might consider referral to an endodontist.

The AAE Endodontic Case Difficulty Assessment Form is designed to aid the practitioner in determining appropriate case disposition. The American Association of Endodontists neither expressly nor implicitly warrants any positive results associated with the use of this form. This form may be reproduced but may not be amended or altered in any way.

AAE Endodontic Case Difficulty Assessment Form

Criteria and Subcriteria	Minimal Difficulty	Moderate Difficulty	High Difficulty
A. PATIENT CONSIDERATIONS			
Medical history	☐ No medical problem (ASA Class 1*)	☐ One or more medical problems (ASA Class 2*)	☐ Complex medical history/serious illness/disability (ASA Classes 3-5*)
Anesthesia	☐ No history of anesthesia problems	☐ Vasoconstrictor intolerance	☐ Difficulty achieving anesthesia
Patient disposition	☐ Cooperative and compliant	☐ Anxious but cooperative	☐ Uncooperative
Ability to open mouth	☐ No limitation	☐ Slight limitation in opening	☐ Significant limitation in opening
Gag reflex	☐ None	☐ Gags occasionally with radiographs/treatment	☐ Extreme gag reflex which has compromised past dental care
Emergency condition	☐ Minimum pain or swelling	☐ Moderate pain or swelling	☐ Severe pain or swelling
B. DIAGNOSTIC AND TREATMENT CONSIDERATIONS			
Diagnosis	☐ Signs and symptoms consistent with recognized pulpal and periapical conditions	☐ Extensive differential diagnosis of usual signs and symptoms required	☐ Confusing and complex signs and symptoms: difficult diagnosis ☐ History of chronic oral/facial pain
Radiographic difficulties	☐ Minimal difficulty obtaining/interpreting radiographs	☐ Moderate difficulty obtaining/interpreting radiographs (*e.g.*, high floor of mouth, narrow or low palatal vault, presence of tori)	☐ Extreme difficulty obtaining/interpreting radiographs (*e.g.*, superimposed anatomical structures)
Position in the arch	☐ Anterior/premolar ☐ Slight inclination (<10°) ☐ Slight rotation (<10°)	☐ 1st molar ☐ Moderate inclination (10-30°) ☐ Moderate rotation (10-30°)	☐ 2nd or 3rd molar ☐ Extreme inclination (>30°) ☐ Extreme rotation (>30°)
Tooth isolation	☐ Routine rubber dam placement	☐ Simple pretreatment modification required for rubber dam isolation	☐ Extensive pretreatment modification required for rubber dam isolation
Morphologic aberrations of crown	☐ Normal original crown morphology	☐ Full coverage restoration ☐ Porcelain restoration ☐ Bridge abutment ☐ Moderate deviation from normal tooth/root form (*e.g.*, taurodontism, microdens) ☐ Teeth with extensive coronal destruction	☐ Restoration does not reflect original anatomy/alignment ☐ Significant deviation from normal tooth/root form (*e.g.*, fusion, dens in dente)
Canal and root morphology	☐ Slight or no curvature (<10°) ☐ Closed apex (<1 mm in diameter)	☐ Moderate curvature (10-30°) ☐ Crown axis differs moderately from root axis. Apical opening 1-1.5 mm in diameter	☐ Extreme curvature (>30°) or S-shaped curve ☐ Mandibular premolar or anterior with 2 roots ☐ Maxillary premolar with 3 roots ☐ Canal divides in the middle or apical third ☐ Very long tooth (>25 mm) ☐ Open apex (>1.5 mm in diameter)
Radiographic appearance of canal(s)	☐ Canal(s) visible and not reduced in size	☐ Canal(s) and chamber visible but reduced in size ☐ Pulp stones	☐ Indistinct canal path ☐ Canal(s) not visible
Resorption	☐ No resorption evident	☐ Minimal apical resorption	☐ Extensive apical resorption ☐ Internal resorption ☐ External resorption
C. ADDITIONAL CONSIDERATIONS			
Trauma history	☐ Uncomplicated crown fracture of mature or immature teeth	☐ Complicated crown fracture of mature teeth ☐ Subluxation	☐ Complicated crown fracture of immature teeth ☐ Horizontal root fracture ☐ Alveolar fracture ☐ Intrusive, extrusive or lateral luxation ☐ Avulsion
Endodontic treatment history	☐ No previous treatment	☐ Previous access without complications	☐ Previous access with complications (*e.g.*, perforation, non-negotiated canal, ledge, separated instrument) ☐ Previous surgical or nonsurgical endodontic treatment completed
Periodontal-endodontic condition	☐ None or mild periodontal disease	☐ Concurrent moderate periodontal disease	☐ Concurrent severe periodontal disease ☐ Cracked teeth with periodontal complications ☐ Combined endodontic/periodontic lesion ☐ Root amputation prior to endodontic treatment

*American Society of Anesthesiologists (ASA) Classification System

Class 1: No systemic illness. Patient healthy.
Class 2: Patient with mild degree of systemic illness, but without functional restrictions, *e.g.*, well-controlled hypertension.
Class 3: Patient with severe degree of systemic illness which limits activities, but does not immobilize the patient.
Class 4: Patient with severe systemic illness that immobilizes and is sometimes life threatening.
Class 5: Patient will not survive more than 24 hours whether or not surgical intervention takes place.

www.asahq.org/clinical/physicalstatus.htm

University-based studies on endodontic outcome have shown overall success rates to be around 90%. However, cross-sectional, retrospective population studies have revealed success rates in only 60% to 75% of cases. It has been shown that there is a consistent association in the cross-sectional studies between poor quality of the root fillings and the presence of a periapical radiolucency. However, several epidemiologic studies have demonstrated that many pretreatment, intratreatment, and post-treatment factors may influence the prognosis of root canal treatment.

Factors Affecting the Prognosis of Endodontic Therapy

Pretreatment factors

Pretreatment factors presented in the literature that may influence the prognosis of endodontic therapy include: age, gender, general health, tooth location, pulp status, symptoms, size of the lesion, and periodontal conditions. However, only the presence of apical periodontitis has been demonstrated to influence the treatment outcome, leading to a 10% to 25% lower success rate than if it were not present preoperatively. Poorer treatment outcome in teeth with apical periodontitis highlights the difference between prevention (which is a challenge of asepsis) and treatment (which is a challenge of disinfection) of an established disease. Poorer outcome may also reflect a lack of understanding as to the importance of disinfection of the root canal before it is filled. We are confident that the prognosis of teeth with and without pretreatment apical periodontitis will be equally high if the suggested protocol described in this manual is followed.

In retreatment cases, pretreatment apical periodontitis is clearly demonstrated to be even more detrimental to the treatment outcome, thereby highlighting the difficulty in disinfecting the root canals of previously treated teeth.

Treatment-related factors

Several treatment-related factors may influence the prognosis of endodontic treatment, including apical extent of root canal filling, apical enlargement, number of treatment sessions, materials and techniques used, and treatment complications. Extrusion of filling materials beyond the root end generally results in a poorer treatment outcome in cases with periapical inflammation, but it does not compromise teeth with a healthy apical periodontium. It is observed that in infected canals, a root filling that is shorter than 1 mm from the radiographic apex results in a less favorable prognosis than one that is filled 0.5 to 1 mm from the radiographic apex. In noninfected cases, root canal fillings 0 to 2 mm from the radiographic apex have similarly high outcomes. Also, the use of a calcium hydroxide intracanal medicament in teeth with apical periodontitis appears to result in a higher incidence of healing. Some studies have demonstrated a higher success rate (about 9%) for treatments using the

Treatment Outcome and Prognosis of Endodontic Therapy

- Vital and necrotic pulps without periapical lesions: 90–98%
- Nonvital pulps with periapical lesions: 80–90%, drop to 50–60% with bad endodontic quality
- Retreatment of teeth without periapical lesions: 89–96%
- Retreatment of teeth with periapical lesions: 60–74%

Fig 5-1

modified step-back technique. Moreover, it appears that different sealants may influence the prognosis of the treatment. Treatment complications, such as perforations in the furcation area, file separations, and sealant extrusion, may contribute to a surprisingly small proportion (4%) of endodontic treatment failures.

Post-treatment factors

It has become increasingly clear that coronal microleakage following endodontic therapy may lead to root canal infection and subsequent failure. The coronal restoration will protect the root canal filling material and provide an additional barrier to re-infection of the root canal space. In cases where the canal is filled with gutta-percha and sealant, the coronal restoration may be more effective (and thus more important) than the root filling in preventing coronal microleakage.

During the past 80 years, numerous studies have been published on the prognosis and treatment outcome of endodontic therapy. Most of these studies vary considerably in material composition, treatment procedures, and methodology, which makes it difficult to compare them and form solid conclusions. Nevertheless, the information accumulated from these studies provides insight into the outcome of endodontic therapy (Fig 5-1). The following general conclusions can be made:

- The prognosis of endodontic therapy, when performed optimally, is extremely good.
- Reasons for failure of endodontic treatment are almost always infection in the root canal space and its influence on the periapical tissues.
- Endodontic infection is often associated with inadequate root canal instrumentation and root canal filling, and/or inadequate coronal restoration.

Treatment Follow-up

Failures following endodontic therapy do occur. Thus, clinical-radiographic follow-up examinations should take place 6 and 12 months after completion of the treatment. If necessary, the period of observation can be extended up to 4 years, especially in cases of apical periodontitis.

Suggested Reading

1. American Association of Endodontists website (http:\\www.aae.org).
2. Friedman S. Prognosis of initial endodontic therapy. Endodont Topics 2002;2:59–88.
3. Tronstad L. Clinical endodontics. 2nd ed. Stuttgart: Thieme, 2003:247–249.

Index

F

G

H

I

M

N

O

P

R

S

T

V

W